The Yoga Beginner's Bible

Top 63 Illustrated Poses for Weight Loss, Stress Relief and Inner Peace

Copyright © 2015 by Tai Morello

Table of Contents

Introduction

From the outside yoga can seem like an esoteric, mystical endeavor exclusively reserved to Tibetan monks and spiritual adepts. This could not be further from the truth. Yoga is not only accessible to anyone, it is easy to learn if you have the right mindset and the benefits are only a few minutes away.

In fact, several studies have confirmed that a single yoga class for inpatients at a psychiatric hospital had the ability to significantly reduce tension, anxiety, depression, anger, hostility, and fatigue.

In this book you will learn why many highly successful people like Robert Downey Jr, Jennifer Aniston and Russel Brand set aside time off their busy schedules to engage in the life-changing practice of yoga.

This book will show you how to instill simple yoga techniques into your daily routine, inevitably leading you to a healthier, happier and more successful life.

The Yoga Beginner's Bible will show you how to instill simple yoga techniques into your daily routine, inevitably leading you to a healthier, happier and more successful life. You will discover how yoga can have profound effects not just on your body, but on virtually every aspect of your life – your mind, relationships, health and even your career.

What is Yoga?

Before we get into the practical how-to of various yogic poses, we should consider what it is we're actually talking about and what it's for. Yoga has been practiced in India for thousands of years. The word *yoga* comes from Sanskrit and is related to the English word *yoke*. Just as a yoke joins an ox to a cart or a plow, *yoga* joins mind and body together in a well-integrated union. On a spiritual level, yoga unites the individual's personal experience to an experience of the absolute reality.

Yoga refers to a broad variety of ancient Indian spiritual practices. These practices are designed to liberate the individual from their ordinary, bound, unfree experience of the self and the world, into an expansive, unlimited state of complete freedom.

So right away we can do away with the idea that, in order to do yoga, you need to sign up with a religious group and give up your own beliefs, adopting a new set of doctrines and strange behaviors. If you're not into the metaphysical ideas behind yoga as spiritual transformation, that's no problem. Yoga is, first and foremost, *personal, practical*, and *experiential*. What you get out of it depends on what you bring into it; your goals and purposes for doing yoga will determine what kind of positive effect it has on your life.

In particular, the popular perception associates yoga with a system of bendy, twisty physical movements and positions. Some may even think yoga is just glorified stretching. But yoga is about more than just stretching. It's about creating balance in body and mind, and joining the two together and bringing them into close communication.

Recent scientific research into the effects of yoga on the body and mind have shown that these physical practices have enormous benefits for physical and psychological health. They can help you lose weight, tone muscles, treat a number of medical problems, improve your flexibility and posture, keep your muscles relaxed and supple, regulate your appetite, etc. They also decrease the all-too-common psychological sufferings of stress, anxiety, and depression, improve concentration and mindfulness, and boost your mood and brainpower overall.

Yoga offers a profound sense of physical and psychological wellbeing. Through the practice of yoga, your body and mind will become more and more closely integrated. That's the central lesson of yoga: by connecting with our bodies more deeply, we go further into our experience as embodied beings in the world. That, in turn, will enrich our lives, as we bring the mindful awareness of yoga into our everyday world.

Finally, a word of warning needs to be said about the practices that follow. Some yoga poses can be dangerous if you're not careful. You can get injured trying to get into some positions. So proceed with caution. Always pay attention to what your body is telling you, and don't do anything if it star. to feel uncomfortable or painful. Sometimes your body will w. sper, "Um, maybe not." Sometimes it will scream, "NO WAY, . TOP NOW!" Be careful and sensitive to these messages.

While this book is intended to give you an introduction to the physical poses and the meditative side of yoga, it's strongly advised that you learn yoga under the guidance of a qualified and experienced instructor. A good yoga teacher can help you avoid mistakes and injury, correct your posture, and guide you into more advanced stages of practice as you get deeper and deeper into yoga.

Yoga Poses for Optimal Health

This chapter is divided into several sections. The first section is on the *Surya Namaskara* sequence of poses, which is one of the most famous and important practices of yoga. The poses in surya namaskara have many benefits for the body and mind, improving stress, mood, promoting weight loss and muscle tone, and helping to relieve many common illnesses and conditions. Because of *surya namaskara* is such a powerful way to promote overall health, it has its own dedicated section.

The other sections of the chapter divide the positions according to different goals of practice. There is a section for weight loss and toning the muscles, a section for various therapeutic applications, from relieving back problems to reducing anxiety and depression. Many poses do not just benefit one area, but here they're organized according to their primary benefits.

Surya Namaskara / Sun Salutations Group

The asanas in this group form one of the most popular, core practices of yoga. The name comes from *surya*, the sun, and *namaskara*, expressing homage or greeting. The asanas in this group have many physical benefits and also double as a way of honoring the positive, life-giving light of the sun. Through *surya namaskara*, the practitioner internalizes the sun's beneficial, vitalizing energy, enlivening his or her body, mind, and spirit.

Scientific research corroborates the traditional wisdom on *surya namaskara*'s benefits. Even if you perform no other positions, ten or twenty minutes of *surya namaskara* every day will reduce stress and increase your overall physical health. Researchers have found a difference between performing this sequence slowly and quickly. The advantage of going through the positions several times quickly is similar to other aerobic exercises and improves cardiovascular and respiratory health. It has tremendous overall benefits, promotes weight loss, improves digestion, strengthens the abdominal muscles, reduces stress and anxiety, increases flexibility, tones the muscles in the arms and legs, strengthens the back, makes you look young, and, for women, promotes a regular menstrual cycle.

There are twelve poses to be performed as part of a single sequence—seven initial poses, which are then repeated in reverse, coming back to the original pose. You'll see what this means as we go through the poses one by one and learn how they all flow together.

1. Pranamasana / Prayer Pose

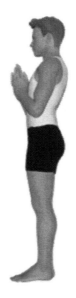

Begin by standing with the feet together. The back, neck, and head should be held straight, so that your entire body is aligned. Join the palms of your hands at the level of your heart in a gesture of respect. Breathe normally, in a relaxed way. Allow any tension in the body to relax, and feel the weight of your body where your feet touch the ground. Gently follow the breath as it goes in and out, just allowing your attention to rest on the the movements of the breath. You may close your eyes or keep them open, maintaining a gentle gaze and looking ahead.

Pranamasana establishes a restful, meditative mindset at the beginning of your session. It induces relaxation and brings your concentration within, allowing you to feel calm and centered.

Benefits: *Pranamasana* relaxes the mind, enhances focus, and gives a sense of balance to body and mind.

2. *Hasta Uttanasana / Raised Arms Pose*

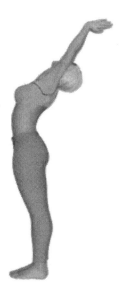

From the standing position of prayer pose, raise both arms high above your head as you inhale. The arms should be separated, held apart at shoulder width. Arch your arms, head, and torso backwards in a gentle curve, so that you feel the muscles in your abdomen stretching.

Benefits: This pose stretches and tones the abdominal muscles. It engages and strengthens muscles in the arms, shoulders, and back. Specifically, this helps improve various spinal problems and stiffness and tension in the shoulders and back. *Hasta uttanasana* increases lung capacity by expanding the ribcage and opening up the chest. It also improves digestion by stretching abdominal organs.

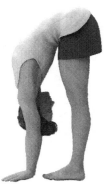

As you exhale, bend forward and touch the floor with the fingers or palms of your hands on either side of your feet. Do not bend your knees: keep your legs straight. If you can, touch your knees with your head. But this will be a challenge to accomplish at first, and you may even have difficulty bringing your hands all the way to the floor.

It is important to remember, in this as in every yoga position, not to try to force your body into a position that it does not want to hold. Yoga is not about the mechanical repetition of positions. It is about bringing the mind and body into harmony with one another. As your mind becomes more and more attuned to your body, you will become aware of the messages that the body is communicating to you. If you experience any pain or strain while attempting a position, that means your body is sending you a clear signal: *No, don't force it, ease up a bit.* So listen to these messages and don't push yourself any farther than is comfortable. If you can't make it all the way, just bend forward as far as you can go and no farther. In time, your flexibility will improve.

Benefits: *Padahastasana* stretches and lengthens the muscles in your back and legs, especially your hamstrings. It allows your shoulders and neck to relax. It also benefits the wrists and can improve the symptoms of carpal tunnel syndrome. It improves digestion by targeting abdominal problems and can help relieve constipation. It also improves circulation.

4. Ashva Sanchalanasana / Equestrian Pose

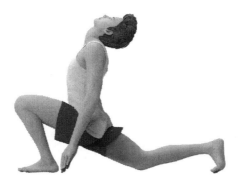

From hands-to-feet pose, with the palms of your hands on the floor, stretch your right leg back as far as it can go while inhaling. Simultaneously bend your left knee without moving your left foot from its position. Bend your back and neck, so that the head is arched backwards and your eyes gaze directly above you. As you achieve the final position, your fingertips should remain touching the floor, shoulder-width apart on either side of your left foot.

Benefits: This position stretches, strengthens, and improves flexibility in the leg muscles. It stretches the abdominal organs, stimulating their functioning.

5. Adho Mukha Svanasana / Downward-Facing Dog Pose

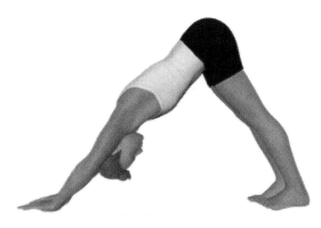

From equestrian pose, bring the left foot back and place it beside the right foot as you exhale. At the same time, straighten your arms and legs and push your butt up towards the ceiling. Lower your head between your arms, so that your ears are aligned with your inner arm. Press the heels of your feet to the floor. Take some time to breathe deeply and let yourself feel the stretch in your calves, thighs, shoulders, and arms.

Again, it is important not to force yourself into position, so as to avoid injury. Get your body as close as it can comfortably get into downward-facing dog, and no closer.

Benefits: Downward-facing dog stretches the legs, arms, shoulders, and spine, strengthening the muscles there. By pressing the heels to the ground, you stretch the calf muscles, which can benefit conditions such as tendinitis of the foot. It improves digestion and the immune system and stimulates circulation. The downward position of the head increases blood flow to the sinuses. It also energizes the body and mind and helps reduce stress.

6. Ashtanga Namaskara / Eight-point Salutation

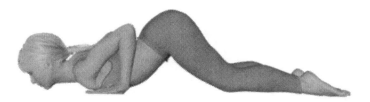

This position is so called because eight parts of the body touch the floor and the body is positioned as if prostrating. From downward-facing dog, lower yourself to the floor so that your knees, chest, hands, and chin are all touching the floor. The toes are bent, resting on the floor. Your butt and abdomen should be raised into the air, and your shoulders touch the backs of your hands. The eyes look forward.

When you move into *ashtanga namaskara*, there is no inhaling or exhaling. Instead, hold the breath outside for a few seconds as you maintain this position—that is, move into eight-point salutation from downward-facing dog *after* exhaling.

Benefits: The eight-point salutation strengthens the muscles in the arms, legs, and chest, and helps loosen up the upper part of the spine, flexing the neck and the area between the shoulder blades.

7. Bhujangasana / Cobra Pose

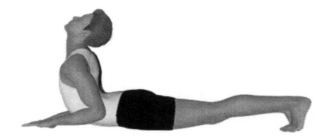

Lower your hips to the floor. As you inhale, straighten your arms somewhat but keep them slightly bent. Arch your back and lift your chest from the floor. Bend your head back, gazing upwards with your eyes. Only lift your chest and arch your back as far as they can go without lifting your hips and pelvic area from the floor; unless your spine is very flexible, your elbows will probably remain somewhat bent. The feet may be either lie flat on the floor, or balance on bent toes. Squeeze your buttocks to remove pressure from your lower back.

Benefits: Cobra pose increases flexibility in the spine, helping to relieve stiffness in the lower back especially. It stretches the muscles in your chest and abdomen. It stimulates abdominal organs, in particular improving digestion and helping to alleviate constipation. It elevates your mood and relieves stress. For women, it helps promote regular menstruation.

Contraindications: If you have spinal problems or pain in your back, you may find this position a bit uncomfortable or painful, so don't try to force yourself into it. Take it easy on spine, keeping your elbows bent, and do not arch your back to the point of discomfort.

8. Adho Mukha Svanasana / Downward-Facing Dog Pose

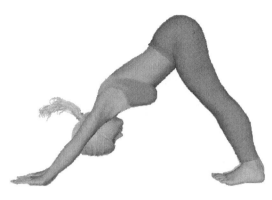

As you exhale, resume downward-facing dog just as before, once again lifting your buttocks towards the ceiling, pushing your heels to the floor, and lowering your head between your arms. Starting with step 8, you will be performing the same sequence *in reverse*, so the positions will be the same as described above.

9. Ashva Sanchalanasana / Equestrian Pose

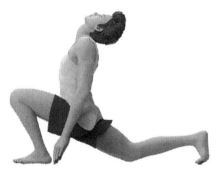

From downward-facing dog, bend your left leg and bring it forward so that the foot rests between your hands. Resume the equestrian pose as before, with your left leg forward and your right leg stretched back. (When you repeat the entire twelve-position sequence, you will alter (4) and (9) by keeping your right leg forward and your left leg stretched back.)

10. *Padahastasana / Hands-to-Feet Pose*

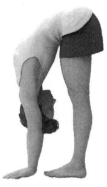

As you exhale, bend your right leg and bring it forward so that it rests next to your left. Straighten your knees and keep your hands on the floor next to your legs, resuming *padahastasana* as before.

11. *Hasta Uttanasana / Raised Arms Pose*

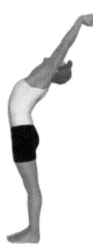

As you inhale, resume *hasta uttanasana* as before, straightening your body and lifting your arms high above your head and arching your back and neck.

12. Pranamasana / Prayer Pose

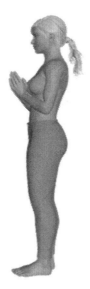

As you exhale, straighten your back and bring your arms down, holding your hands, palms pressed together, in a gesture of respect.

That completes the first half of the sequence of *surya namaskara*. From the prayer pose, let your arms hang by your side and just allow your muscles to relax as you stand, breathing deeply and focusing your mind on the soothing rhythms of the breath. Then resume the prayer pose and go through all twelve positions a second time, this time with the right foot forward instead of the left as you perform the equestrian pose in steps (4) and (9).

You can perform all twenty-four steps of *surya namaskara* once or several times, depending on how much time you have and how much benefit you want to get out of it. In the beginning, it is probably wise to keep the number of repetitions in the range of one to three as your body gets used to it. When you are finished, you can let your body rest in the corpse pose or *shavasana*, to allow your breathing and heartbeat to relax and your mind to rest freely. Corpse pose is described in the chapter on resting positions.

Surya namaskara can be performed quickly and slowly, depending on your purpose. If you go through the sequence slowly, then hold each position for fifteen to thirty cycles of the breath, allowing your muscles and mind to relax fully. Doing *surya namaskara* slowly has profound benefits for relaxing body and mind and induces a deep meditative state and heightened awareness of the body. In addition to developing meditative awareness and integration of body and mind, this can also have a tremendous effect on reducing stress and anxiety, alleviating depression, and regulating your mood, which will help you remain calm and happy throughout the day.

Performed quickly, *surya namaskara* is a powerful cardiovascular workout that strengthens muscles in the entire body, improves respiratory and circulatory function, and promotes weight loss, in addition to the specific physical benefits of each position. It goes without saying that a healthy amount of exercise is also a huge mood boost, and also helpful for reducing stress. But in general, we could say that going through the sequence slowly has meditative and mental benefits, while going quickly benefits the body.

Chandra Namaskara

In addition to the sequence of poses in Surya Namaskara, you might also find it very positive to practice *chandra namaskara*—a.k.a. moon salutations. Sun salutations develop the warming, active, masculine, solar energy of body and mind, while practicing moon salutations cultivates the feminine, lunar aspect, which is cooling and gentle. Sun salutations relate to the energy of the right or *pingala* channel of the subtle energy network of the body, while moon salutations are work more with the energy of the *ida* channel on the left side of the body. I talk about this in more detail in my books on chakras and kundalini.

Adding chandra namaskara to your yoga practice makes it balanced. If you only practice sun salutations without balancing it with moon salutations, there may be something kind of off or one-sided about your practice of yoga.

The sequence of chandra namaskara is the same as sun salutations, except that there is an extra pose *after* the equestrian pose in steps 4 and 9. Hence it has fourteen poses in all, which are connected to the fourteen days of the waxing and waning modes of the moon. The extra pose in chandra namaskara is *ardha chandrasana,* or half moon pose.

4b, 9b. Ardha Chandrasana / Half Moon Pose

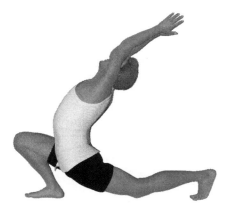

In equestrian pose, one leg is bent forward while the other is extended behind you. Your fingers touch the floor and your back and neck are arched upwards.

The position of the body is mostly the same here. From equestrian pose, lift your hands from the floor and bring your palms together in front of your chest. Then stretch the arms high above your head and arch them backwards. Hold that position briefly, then again bring the fingers down to the floor in equestrian pose before proceeding to the next pose in the sequence.

Just as with sun salutations, moon salutations are best done at the beginning of your practice. While the ideal time to practice sun salutations is in the morning at dawn, or when the sun is low in the sky, moon salutations are best practiced in the evening, in the light of the moon. The best time to do moon salutations is during the full moon.

Joint-Loosening Poses

If you're brand new to yoga, some of the more stretchy and bendy poses can be intimidating. Rather than get put off by the challenge, you might want to ease into yoga by starting with some exercises to loosen your joints. These exercises target some of the areas that are most commonly stiff to make them more pliable for the rest of your yoga practice.

You can start off by performing only the joint-loosening exercises. Or, if you feel like you're ready to jump in but still think you can benefit from loosening up a bit, you can put them at the beginning of your yoga session, before *Surya namaskara*.

Griva Sanchalana / Neck Rotation

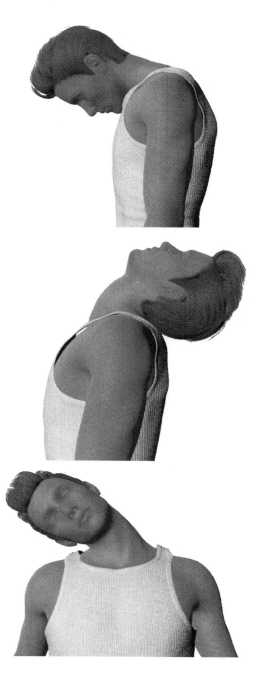

Sit on the floor. You may sit with your legs stretched out in front of you, or cross-legged. For the purposes of this exercise, it doesn't make much difference.

Let your head hang forward as far as possible, but keep your back straight. Just relax your neck muscles and let your chin drop as far as it can.

Rotate your head clockwise, slowly. If you feel some stiffness in your neck, go even slower and try to relax your neck muscles as much as possible. You will bring your head from the forward position to a position where it's bent back, then again to the forward position.

As your head goes from front to back, breathe in. Then, as it goes from back to the original position, breathe out. Repeat this rotating movement seven times, then stop when your head is in the forward position.

Repeat, going counterclockwise. Keep the same breathing pattern. Again do it seven times.

Benefits: Stiffness in the neck is such a common problem that results from long periods of sitting at work, or the position we find ourselves in when we sleep. This loosens the neck and relieves stiffness and tension. It will also make it possible to perform more advanced yoga movements.

Skandha Chakra / Shoulder Rotation

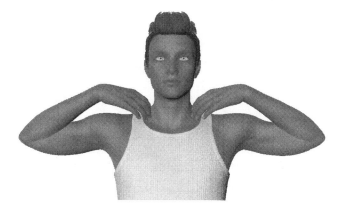

The next area to target is the shoulders, another common problem area due to stress, bad posture from a desk job, and so on. Sit as you did before during the neck rotation.

Keep your back straight throughout this exercise. Touch your shoulders with your fingers. Then rotate both arms. Bring the elbows around in a big circle. In the upstroke, try to touch your elbows to each other. On the downstroke, allow the backs of your hands to brush your ears. Breathe in when moving up and out when moving down.

Do this seven times, then reverse direction, repeating seven times more.

Benefits: In addition to relieving common shoulder tension, this movement opens up the shoulders and straightens them, correcting the common slumped, rounded, or slouched posture many people carry.

Manibandha Chakra / Wrist Rotation

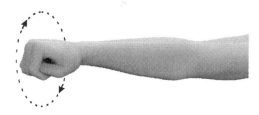

Sit as you did in the previous two exercises. Stretch both arms in front of you, parallel to the ground, and make two fists. Then rotate your wrists in a circular motion. Make sure you keep your arms perfectly straight, without moving your elbows. Within that limited range, try to move your wrists as much as possible.

Do seven rotations, then change direction and repeat in the other way.

Benefits: In addition to loosening up your wrists for more advanced positions, this will help to relieve pain and injury from long periods of typing, etc., such as carpal tunnel syndrome.

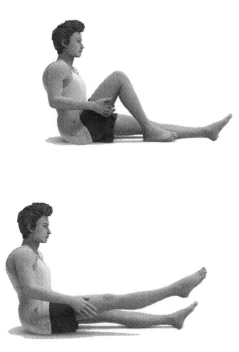

Sit with your legs extended in front of you, flat on the floor, and your back straight. Pull your left knee in, grasping the inside of your thigh beneath the knee with both hands. Let your foot hover above the floor without touching it. Then stretch it out again.

Repeat seven rounds with your left leg, then do it all again with your right leg.

Benefits: Knee pain and knee injuries are exceedingly common, so the purpose of this exercise is to give some work to the knees, making them more supple, relieving any stiffness, and increasing flexibility and range of motion.

Poses for Weight Loss & Muscle Tone

In addition to *surya namaskara*, there are many other yoga poses that promote weight loss and muscle tone. It is hard to single out just a few poses for this category, as weight loss is one of the many benefits of yoga in general, but I have selected a few that are especially good for shedding extra pounds. If you add these to a vigorous, fast-paced practice of *surya namaskara*, you'll be well on your way to losing weight, looking fit, and achieving overall mental and physical wellbeing.

Tadasana / Palm Tree Pose

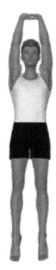

Stand with your feet together or slightly apart and find your balance, arms hanging loosely by your side. Raise your arms overhead and interlock your fingers, turning your palms upward so they face the ceiling. Then lower your hands until your knuckles are resting on the top of our head.

Look forward at a fixed point in front of you and do not move your gaze from this spot. As you inhale, stretch your arms high above you, pulling your shoulder and chest upward with them. Push yourself up on tiptoes, and stretch the whole body in that position, maintaining balance and stability while holding your breath for a few moments.

Then lower the heels and bring your hands back down to their resting position on top of your head, while exhaling. Do five or more rounds, taking a few moments to rest between each round.

Benefits: Palm tree pose stretches the spinal column and can even increase your height. It strengthens muscles in the core, toning the abdominal and back muscles and improving the overall balance of the body. It also strengthens and tones muscles in the arms and legs.

For a variation of this position, once you have achieved good stability and balance in *tadasana,* try taking four steps forward and backward while balancing on your toes.

Tiryana Tadasana / Swaying Palm Tree Pose

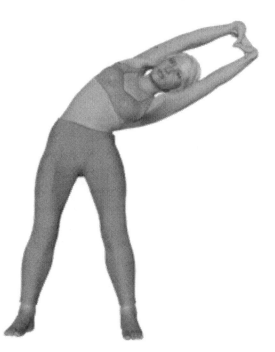

Stand with your feet about two feet apart. With your arms lowered, interlock your fingers and turn the palms outward. As you inhale, raise the arms above your head, as in *tadasana*. Then exhale and bend the body to the left without twisting your abdomen or moving forward or backward. Hold the breath for a few seconds without inhaling. Then, as you straighten out and resume the upright position, breathe in again.

Now repeat the bending movement, only this time bend the body to the right side while exhaling. Again hold that position for a few seconds without breathing in. Then inhale again as you resume a straightened position. Finally, exhale as you lower your arms again. Rest for a moment. Then perform several more rounds, as many as five to ten in total.

Benefits: Swaying palm tree pose strengthens the oblique muscles, toning them and removing love handles. It engages the hard-to-reach muscles that cover the rib cage. It adds overall balance to your core, improving the stability of your posture. It also stretches the spine, relieving minor back injuries such as slipped disc. It also stimulates digestion and relieves constipation.

Once you have stability and flexibility with this posture, you can try doing it while standing on your toes as in *tadasana*.

Ekapada Pranamasana / One-Legged Prayer Pose

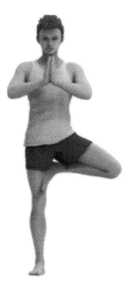

Stand straight with your legs together and your arms hanging loosely. Bend your right knee and grasp the ankle with your right hand. Tuck the sole of your foot on the inside of the left thigh. Bring your heel close to your perineum. Do this slowly, and make sure you have your balance before you proceed.

Bring your hands in front of your just in *anjali mudra*, the gesture of prayer. Hold that position for a minute or two – or for as long as you can keep your balance.

Then relax, bring your right foot to the floor, and do it again with the left foot this time.

Benefits: Strengthens and tones the leg muscles. Stretches the groin and inner thighs. Helps to improve your sense of balance. This pose also encourages energetic harmony between the channels on either side of your body.

Kati Chakrasana / Waist-Rotating Pose

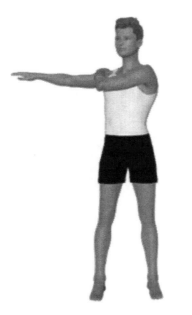

Stand with your feet about one and a half feet apart, with your arms by your side. As you inhale, raise your arms up so that they spread out on either side of you, parallel to the floor. Then, while exhaling, twist your torso around to your left, bringing your right hand to rest on your left shoulder and wrapping your left arm all the away around the back so that the left hand rests on the right waist. Twist your head as far to the left as you can without straining, taking care to make sure that your neck and posture are straight and upright. Hold the breath for several seconds, stretching your abdomen and allowing the muscles to relax. Don't allow your feet to lift from the ground while twisting.

Then inhale as you resume the initial position, and repeat the twist, this time turning to your right. Again hold the breath, and again inhale as you resume the initial position.

Complete at least five rounds. The movements should be performed smoothly, without any sudden movements or jerkiness. For more of a workout, twist left and right at a faster pace.

Benefits: Waist-rotating pose stretches and tones the muscles in the waist, back, and hips. It also loosens up the arms and shoulders. Taken together with palm tree pose and swaying palm tree pose, waist-rotating pose forms the third part of a sequence that can be performed at any time of the day when one is feeling tired or stiff. This threefold sequence is especially useful for office workers who have to sit for long hours, as it loosens up the spine, elevates depressed mood, alleviates stress, and infuses your body and mind with extra energy.

Naukasana / Boat Pose

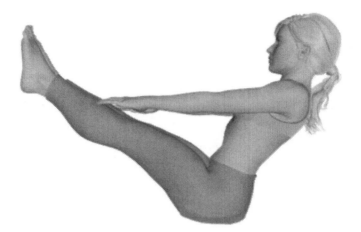

Boat pose is meant to be performed from a supine (lying down) position, and is best performed together with other supine postures. From the supine position, breathe in, then hold the breath as you raise your legs and trunk, together with the shoulders and head, from the ground. Hold the arms straight and parallel to the ground, palms facing down. The whole body should form the shape of a triangle pointing downwards, balanced on the buttocks. Keep your spine straight and gaze at your feet.

Hold this position without breathing for as long as you can—basically, until you need to breathe again. As you return to a supine position (*shavasana*, as described in the relaxation chapter), breathe out again. Allow all the muscles in your body to relax. Then repeat four times, for a total of five rounds.

Benefits: Boat pose exercises your core, especially strengthening and toning the abdominal muscles and helping to remove excess belly fat. It also strengthens and tones muscles in the shoulders, arms, and thighs. It benefits and improves the function of abdominal organs.

Ustrasana / Camel Pose

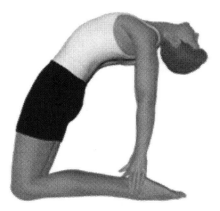

Kneel down on your knees, keeping them hips-width apart, with your back straight and arms hanging by your sides. Keep your feet and knees together. Lean back and grasp one heel with one hand, then the other heel with the other hand. Thrust your stomach forward while keeping your thighs perpendicular to the floor. Arch your back and neck, and bring the head back until you're gazing at the ceiling. Allow some of the weight to fall on your arms and some on your legs, so that the arms support the upper back. Breathe shallowly while in camel pose.

If you're a beginner, you might find it difficult to get into this position. It's worth repeating: Don't force yourself. You might find it easier if you rest on the balls of the feet instead of extending them so that they lie flat on the floor.

Benefits: Camel pose deeply stretches all the muscles in the front of the body, including the neck, chest, abs, thighs, and groin. It is an especially good stretch for the hip flexors. It's also excellent for strengthening the back and improving posture. By stretching the abdominal muscles, it also improves digestion.

Contraindications: Do not try camel pose if you suffer from serious back problems or high blood pressure.

Ardha Halasana / Half Plough Pose

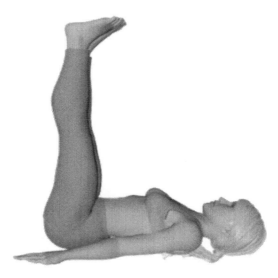

Lie on the back in the supine position with your legs together. While inhaling, left both legs up slowly until they are at a right angle to the floor. Don't lift the buttocks from the floor, but keep them and the back lying flat against the floor. Your abs should be doing the work in this position. Hold this position, and your breath, for several seconds. Then exhale and gently lower your legs to the floor.

That completes one round. It should be repeated for five to ten rounds.

Alternately, you can bring your legs to a forty-five degree angle to your torso. In either case, with your legs held at ninety or forty-five degrees, you can experiment with separating them and bring them back together, and other movements, to reach different abdominal muscles.

Benefits: Half plough pose engages and tones abdominal muscles, removes belly fat, and helps you get closer to achieving a six-pack. It tones the muscles in the thighs and hips, as well. It improves digestion and flatulence.

This is a preliminary position to the more challenging *halasana,* the plough pose, described later on, and should be mastered before trying the latter position.

Dhanurasana / Bow Pose

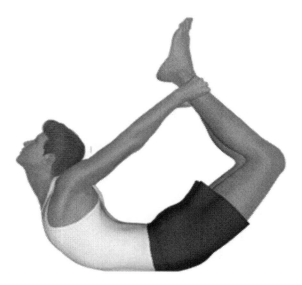

Lie on your stomach with your chin on the floor and your feet hips-width apart. Bend your knees and bring the heels as close as you can to your buttocks. Grasp the ankles with your hands, and, keeping your arms straight, extend the legs so that your chest and knees lift from the floor and the feet move upwards, away from the body. Your abdomen and groin should remain on the floor. Arch your neck so that your eyes are directed upwards. Your legs should be doing the work to hold you in position, allowing the rest of your muscles—back, abs, chest, arm—to relax.

Continue holding this position and breathing for about twenty seconds. Then exhale and gently relax the leg muscles, slowly lowering yourself to the floor. Complete about five rounds.

Benefits: Bow pose strengthens the back and abs and tones muscles in the legs, arms, and chest. It improves your flexibility and decreases stress.

Setu Asana / Bridge Pose

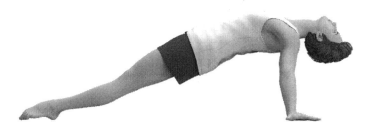

Sit on the floor with your legs extended in front of you. Place your hands, fingers pointing backwards, on the floor about one foot behind you. Keep your elbows straight. You should be leaning backwards slightly.

Inhale, then, holding the breath, lift your waist and torso, so that your feet and hands are touching the ground and the rest of your body is arching upwards. Ideally, the feet should rest flat against the floor. Relax your neck and allow your head to hang loosely.

Hold the position for as long as you are comfortable, then exhale and gently lower your body to the original seated position.

This can be repeated for ten rounds.

Benefits: Bridge pose strengthens and tones the lower back muscles. It also strengthens the arms and legs. It benefits posture, back problems, and stretches the achilles tendon.

Phalakasana / Plank Pose

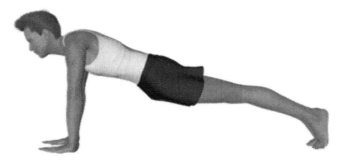

Start by kneeling on the floor, then raise your buttocks so that your thighs are vertical. Lean forward and put your hands on the floor, palms down, beneath your shoulders and at shoulders width. Lift the buttocks up, keeping your knees straight, so that you are balancing on your hands and toes. Keep your buttocks slightly lifted, against the force of gravity that pulls your hips towards the floor and arches your back. Keep your back straight, your neck aligned with your spine so that the eyes are looking towards the floor.

In the final position, you should feel that the muscles in both your back and abdomen are engaged. Maintain this for as long as you can. You may even find that your body starts shaking while you hold this position. If it's too difficult to support the weight on your hands, try lowering yourself on your elbows.

As a variation, from the final position, try lifting each leg alternately until it's parallel to the floor and the weight is distributed to the other foot.

Benefits: Plank pose tones the abdominal and back muscles. It strengthens the arms, shoulders, and wrists. It improves balance.

Vasishtasana / Side Plank Pose

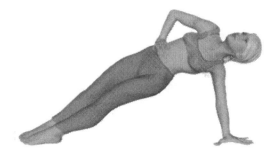

From plank pose, shift onto the side of your right foot, so that your right foot and right hand support the entire weight of your body. Your left foot rests on your right, and the left hand rests on the left hip.

The right arm should not be directly below the shoulder, but a little higher. Keep your back straight, so that your spine is aligned with your legs. Breathe normally.

Alternately, you may find it easier to support your weight on your elbow instead of your hand. In other variations, lift your left arm so that it is vertical. You may also lift your left leg, or even try to hold your left foot with your left hand, while keeping both leg and arm straight.

Perform this pose three times on each side, right and left.

Benefits: Side plank pose strengthens and tones the arms, legs, and lower back, as well as the abdomen. In particular, it targets the oblique muscles, reducing the appearance of love handles.

Utthan Pristhasana / Lizard Pose Version 1

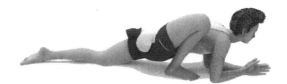

Start in downward-facing dog. Bring your left foot forward a little bit behind your left hand and to the outside. Keep your right leg stretched behind you. Lower your elbows to the floor and rest your forearms entirely on the ground.

Hold for about a minute, then return to downward-facing dog. Then repeat with your right leg forward this time.

If you want some extra stretch, extend your back leg farther behind you in the final position.

Benefits: This is amazing for opening up the hips and stretching the legs, hamstrings, and groin. It strengthens and tones the thighs and opens and shoulders and chest. It prepares for body for more advanced poses that require very flexible hips.

Vipareeta Shalabhasana / "Superman" Pose

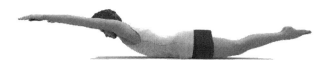

Lie on your stomach with your feet flat against the floor and your arms stretched out in front of you. Bring your palms together.

Breathe in and use your back and abdominal muscles to lift your feet, thighs, chest, arms, and head from the floor. The only part touching the floor should be your belly and groin. Really stretch your arms in front of you and your legs behind you. Your arms and legs should not be bent.

Hold that position for as long as you can, then relax, resting your entire body on the floor.

Benefits: Superman pose is a great way to strengthen your lower back and your abs. It also stretches your arms, legs, shoulders, and chest.

Trikonasana / Triangle Pose

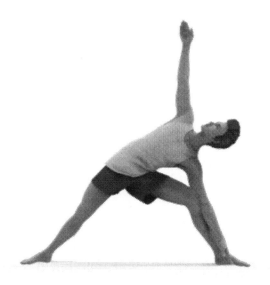

Stand with your feet apart about three feet. As you inhale, raise your arms to either side, holding them parallel to the ground.

Then turn your left foot, pointing it to your left. Exhale and bend your torso to the left, without bending it forward. Bend the left knee slightly. Keeping your arms straight, touch the toes of your left foot with your left hand. Your right arm should be pointing straight up to the sky. Turn your face upwards and rest your gaze on your right hand.

Hold that position for a few seconds without breathing. Then inhale and return to the standing position, arms stretched out to the sides. Repeat the same movement on the right side. Do five to ten rounds.

Once you are comfortable with this pose, try doing it with both legs straight.

Benefits: This position tones the entire body and is good for weight less. It stretches your core. It stretches the legs and arms, as well. It improves digestion and appetite, and alleviates depression. Practiced daily—especially if you do it quickly, with ten or more rounds—it burns stubborn belly fat and will reduce your waistline.

Utthita parsvakonasana / Extended side angle pose

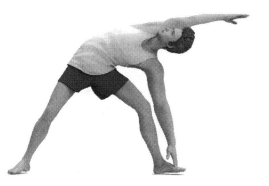

This is a variation of *trikonasana*. In triangle pose, one hand touches the foot, while the other is raised towards the sky. In extended side-angle pose, you take the raised arm and lower it towards your head. The arm points straight past your head, in a direction roughly parallel to the ground. This might be a bit too much of a stretch for your sides at first. Just get it as close as you can. Keep your knee bent. Then to it on the opposite side.

Benefits: The benefits are the same as in trikonasana. This pose gives an extra stretch to your side and tones your obliques. It also stimulates your abdominal organs.

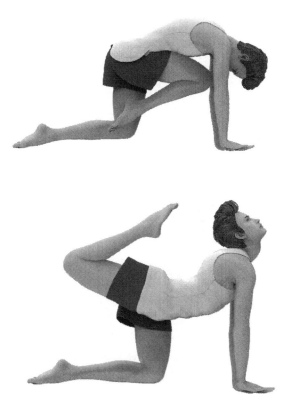

Start with kneeling on the floor, as in marjari asana, than move into the same cat pose. Keep your arms verticle, at 90 degrees to the floor.

Then, as you inhale, extend your left leg behind you, all the way back, lifting it up as far as possible. Bend your left knee and bring your foot towards your head. At the same time, arch your back down and your neck and head up and see if you can touch your toes to your head—but don't strain! Hold that for a few seconds.

Then again extend your left leg. As you inhale, pull it in under you, bending the knee. Bring it towards your chest. Now your back should be arched in the other direction, and your head and neck curving downwards.

Repeat this a few times with the same leg in a swinging motion. Make sure that leg doesn't touch the floor. Then switch to the right leg and do the same thing with that one.

Benefits: Tiger pose targets extra weight in the hips and thighs, burning fat in those areas. It loosens and the muscles in the back and gives a nice stretch to the spine. It benefits the female reproductive organs. It also improves digestion and circulation.

Yoga Poses for Therapeutic Purposes

For Back and Muscle Pain

The following positions can be used to improve back conditions, stretching the spine, loosening muscles in the upper and lower back and shoulders, and remedying injuries such as slipped disc. They also release the tension so often stored in the back, which is a major source of stress.

Marjari Asana / Cat Pose

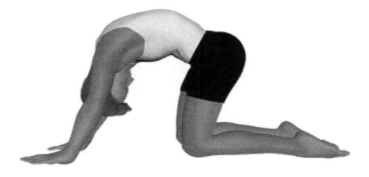

From a kneeling position, lift up your waist so that your thighs are perpendicular to the floor and you are standing on your knees. Lean forward and put your palms on the floor in front of you, as if you are crawling on all fours. Keep your hands aligned with your knees.

Inhale and arch your neck and head upwards. At the same time, press your belly downwards so that your back is bent towards the floor. When breathing in, fill your lungs to capacity. Hold the breath for a few seconds.

Then, as you breathing out, arch your back upwards, stretching the spine, and lower your head between your arms. Again hold the breath for a few seconds, before inhaling and starting the next round. Continue for a up to ten rounds.

Benefits: Cat pose is good for back problems and increases flexibility in the spine and shoulders. It also has a soothing, therapeutic effect on the digestive system.

Paschimottasana / Forward Bending Pose

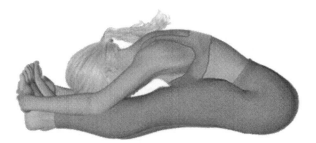

Sit on the floor with your legs extended in front of you, feet together. Exhale slowly and bend forward from the hips, slowly moving your hands along your legs towards your feet. Grab your big toes with your fingers. Relax and breathe in deeply.

Without bending your legs, use your arms to gently pull the head closer to the knees. Don't try to force anything. The back should be relaxed during this movement, which allows the forward motion to gently stretch the back muscles and spine. During this forward pull, inhale again.

Hold this position for some time, continuing to breathe. Then slowly return to the original seated position. You may perform five rounds of this.

Benefits: Forward bending pose deeply stretches the spine along its entire length. It also stretches the hamstrings and increases flexibility in the back and hips. It tones and strengthens the shoulders.

Janu Shirshasana / Head-to-Knee Pose

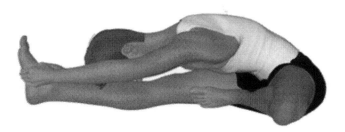

As in forward bending pose, begin seated, with your legs extended in front of you. Bend the left knee and bring the sole of the left foot against the inside of the right thigh. Stretch your hands towards the right foot, bending forward, until they reach the right foot. Grasp the toes with the left hand and the edge of the foot with the right. Bring your head as close as you can to the knee of the right foot.

For beginners, it will be difficult to bring the head all the way to the knee. Don't try to force this! The position should relax the back, while the arms do the work. Hold the final position for as long as is comfortable and breathe deeply.

Then repeat the pose, this time with the other leg. Complete five rounds for each leg.

Benefits: Just like forward-bending pose, it gives a deep stretch to the entire length of the spine, as well as the muscles on each side of the back. It also stretches the legs and makes them more flexible for the meditation positions.

Utthita Janu Shirshasana / Head-Between-Knees Standing Pose

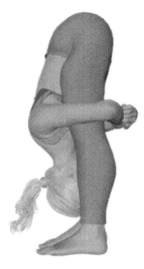

Stand upright with the legs one and a half feet apart. Extend your arms in front of you so they are parallel to the ground. Exhale completely, then hold your breath and bend from your hips. Bring the arms around your legs, and clasp your hands together. Pull your head closer to the knees with your arms, but do not try to force it. This should stretch your upper back and shoulders, including the area between your shoulder blades, as well as your hamstrings. In this final position, keep holding your breath. Keep this for as long as comfortable before releasing it and returning to the initial upright position as you inhale. Perform five rounds.

If you are flexible enough, unclasp your hands and use them to hold your neck. This is a more advanced version of the same pose.

Benefits: This pose stretches the muscles of the upper back, lengthens the spine, and stretches the hamstrings. It also increases flexibility in the hips. By releasing tension from the upper back, it decreases stress and anxiety. The benefits are similar to those of *padahastasana* (hands-to-feet pose) from the *surya namaskara* section, except that this pose gives an extra stretch to the shoulders and muscles in the upper back around the shoulder blades.

Ardha Shalabhasana / Half Locust Pose

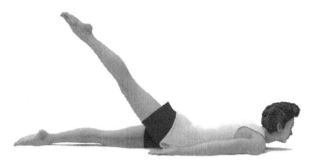

Lie on your stomach. Hold your chin forward and rest it on the floor. Tuck your hands under your thighs, palms down. Then lift your left leg as high as you can without bending it. Your right leg should stay rested on the floor. The arms should provide support, pushing against the ground to give your leg some extra stretch.

Hold that position as long as you can. When you're tired, lower the left leg to the floor. Then repeat with the right leg this time.

You want to keep both legs completely straight throughout this whole pose. Do up to three rounds, then just rest in a prone position, your head turned to the side.

Benefits: This pose strengthens the back and stretches the spine and neck. In addition to strengthening the back muscles, which creates a strong support for the spine, it can also help alleviate slipped disc. Half locust pose will strengthen and prepare you for the more challenging locust pose.

Shalabhasana / Locust Pose

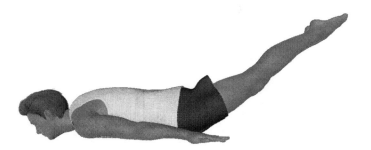

This pose is the same as the previous one, except in this case you lift both legs at the same time. Press with against the floor with your arms to give extra lift to the legs. Again repeat about three times, then simply lie on the floor and rest.

Benefits: The benefits are the same as in half locust pose, but much stronger. This is an excellent way to strengthen your back muscles, so that they become like two columns supporting your spine.

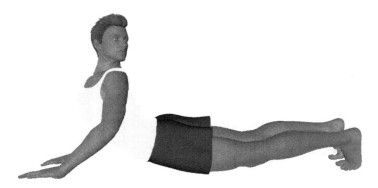

Breathe in and assume the regular cobra pose, but with your feet spread a couple of feet apart. The underside of your toes or balls of your feet should touch the floor. With your eyes, look straight forward; don't arch your head back, as in regular bhujangasana, but hold it perpindicular to the ground.

Holding your breath, turn your head and shoulders to the left and look over your left shoulder at your right foot. Don't try to force it. Just let your back relax. Hold this position briefly, then turn forward again, and twist to the right and hold again for a few seconds.

Again face forward, then exhale as you lower yourself to the ground.

Benefits: This pose has similar benefits to the regular cobra pose (described as part of sun salutations), but gives some extra flexibility to the spine and helps stimulate and soothe the digestive system.

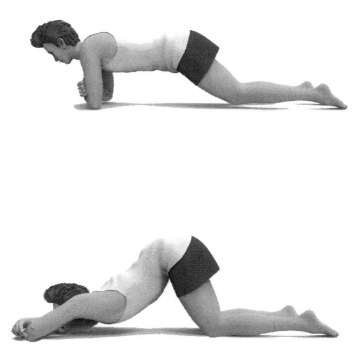

This second "version" of the lizard pose doesn't have much in common with the previous version except for the name.

Lie on your stomach with your arms crossed under your chest. Your hands should clasp the arms above the elbows. Hold the feet slightly apart. Look forward.

Keeping your elbows in place on the floor, raise your body so that you're on your knees and elbows with your torso parallel to the ground.

Then stretch your buttocks backwards and lower your chest to the ground. Rest your chin behind your arms, with your buttocks sticking up in the air. Inhale as you do so.

In one continuous movement, return to the raised position, then lower yourself to the ground as in the beginning. Exhale as you do so.

Benefits: This improves breathing by strengthening the diaphragm, encouraging deep belly breaths. It stretches the shoulder blades and back.

Skandharasana / Shoulder Pose

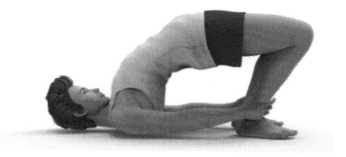

Lie on your back on the floor. Bend your knees and pull your feet up so that the heels touch your buttocks. Then reach down with your arms and hold your ankles.

Now arch your back and lift your butt up off the ground. Imagine a string is pulling you up from the pelvis. In the final position, your thighs should be parallel to the ground and your calves at a right angle. Your shoulders and neck support the weight of your upper body, while the feet take the rest of the weight.

Keep that position for as long as you can, then again return to the original position (with bent knees). Practice for about five rounds.

Benefits: Skandharasana improves your posture and makes your shoulders squarer and stronger. It improves digestion and, in women, encourages healthy menstruation.

Upavistha konasana / Wide-Angle Pose

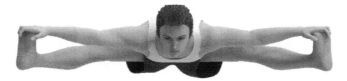

Sit with your legs out in front of you, and lean back slightly on your hands. Spread your legs out to a rough 90-degree angle, or as close as you can get. Press down and lift your butt from the ground and move it forward, so your legs are spread a bit farther apart.

Press your outer thighs against the floor, rotating them a bit. Lift your toes up and stretch the soles of your feet. Putting your hands between your legs, walk them forward slowly as you lean forward. Take it easy here—this gives quite a stretch to your groin, and you don't want to injure yourself!

Lean forward as far as you can without pain or strain, *and no farther.* If you're very flexible, you can lean all the way forward and grab your toes with your fingers. Hold your final position for a minute or two, breathing slowly.

Benefits: Stretches the inside of the legs, the hamstrings, and the groin. This pose also stretches the spine and increases flexibility in the hips.

For the Common Cold

The best yoga practice for relieving symptoms of cold and cough is the *surya namaskara* sequence explained above.

Yoga Pose for Cognitive Benefits and Psychological Health

In general, practicing yoga will decrease stress, anxiety, and depression and give a huge boost to your mood and sense of well-being. But there are a few positions you can do to specifically target this area, as well as enhance your cognitive functioning and increase memory, mental clarity, and intelligence. For these purposes, *surya namaskara,* described above, is excellent. Also good are backward-bending poses, such as bow pose and camel pose, and spine-twisting poses, such as waist-rotating pose and *ardha matsyendrasana* or half spinal twist, described in this section. To that, we can add upside-down poses that increase blood flow to the brain, like *vipareeta karani asana* (inverted pose) and its more advanced version, *sarvangasana* (shoulder stand, not described in this book).

"Seated Twist"

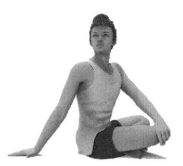

In case Ardha matsyendranasana, or the half spinal twist, is a bit too much for you, you can try this simpler and less demanding "seated twist."

Sit in sukhasana, the comfortable pose. Twist to your left. Put your left hand, palm down, on the floor behind you, while your right hand rests on your left knee. Turn your neck as far as you can without straining, so that you're looking behind you. Hold that pose for twenty counts, breathing slowly and really allowing the muscles in your back, arms, neck, and shoulders to relax.

Then return to sukhasana and repeat on the right side.

Benefits: This is a deeply relaxing position that soothes anxiety and stress. It gives a gentle twist to the spine from the base all the way to the neck, which adds flexibility to the back and improves posture.

Ardha matsyendrasana / Half Spinal Twist

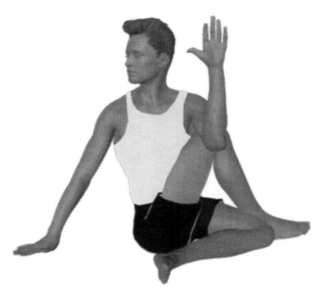

From a seated position, with the legs extended in front of the body, bend the right knee and place the right foot flat on the floor. Bend the left leg and bring the knee under the crook of the right leg, so that the left heel touches the right buttock. Bring the left arm to the right side of the body and to the other side of the right leg, and grasp the right ankle with the left hand. The right leg should be pressing against the left arm.

Keeping the spine straight, exhale and twist your torso to the right, and press your right hand on the floor, elbow locked. Twist your neck to the right as far as is comfortable to add to the twisted position of this pose, but don't allow your shoulders to slouch. Keep your neck straight and upright.

The idea is to use your right leg and left arm to twist the spine without using the back muscles, so that the spine and back muscles are left to relax fully. You should not strain or force anything in this position. Breathe deeply for twenty counts of the breathe, then inhale and slowly return to the starting position.

Then repeat the whole position, this time on the left side.

Benefits: Half spinal twist relieves stress, anxiety, and depression. It helps release deep tension from the back, shoulders, and neck, which often accompanies stress. It is also an excellent back stretch that alternately stretches and contracts the muscles on each side of the back, and can improve back conditions such as slipped disc.

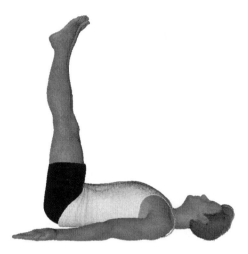

This pose is a preparation for the proper vipareeta karani, in which you raise your legs straight up without support while letting your shoulders take the weight.

In this prepatory pose, place a cushion or two next to a wall. You want to rest your butt and lower back on the pillow, while the legs point straight up and rest against the wall. Your arms and shoulders rest on the floor. Thus your hips will be slightly higher than your chest and shoulders.

Once you're in position, you can simply relax like that and breathe deeply. To return from this asana, bring your knees to your chest, then roll onto your side before getting up.

Benefits: Half inverted pose reverses the usual direction of gravity on the body. Blood will drain from the legs and move to the upper part of the body. The increased blood flow to the brain improves your thinking and cognition in general, as well as bringing relaxation and reducing stress.

If your job or lifestyle is not very active and you sit for long periods of time, this pose is especially helpful. It will help reduce any possible swelling or pain in the legs and feet. It improves circulation overall.

Contraindications: If you have high blood pressure, give this one a pass, as it will increase blood pressure in the upper body.

Vipareeta Karani Asana / Inverted Pose

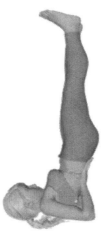

Lie flat on your back with your feet together. Your arms should be at your side, palms against the floor. Inhale while lying down.

Then, holding the breath, lift your legs towards the ceiling and bring them towards your head. Pressing down with your palms, letting the arms do the work, lift your buttocks from the floor, which will cause your back to bend. Lift up the palms but keep the elbows on the floor, then bring the palms against the lower part of your back just below the buttocks to support the weight. If that is too difficult, you can hold your palms against the buttocks. Your elbows and shoulders will support the weight of your body.

Keep your legs at a ninety-degree angle to the floor. Close your eyes and relax, breathing normally for as long as you are comfortable. Then, holding your breath again, bring the knees towards your head again, return your palms face-down to the floor, and slowly lower the buttocks to the floor, finally resting your legs and resuming the original position.

In the beginning, you may find it easier to prop your legs against the wall while holding this position.

Benefits: Inverted pose reverses the force of gravity on the body, which has a number of benefits. In particular, it causes blood flow to the head to increase. The increased blood flow in the brain benefits the mind, relieving anxiety, stress, and depression, improving cognitive functions, and increasing memory and intelligence. Inverted pose also relieves flatulence and hemorrhoids.

Sarpasana / Serpent Pose

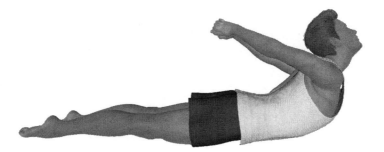

Lie on your stomach with your legs together. Clasp your hands together behind your back, resting them on your buttocks. Rest your chin on the floor.

As you breathe in, raise your chest from the floor as far as you can. Engage your back muscles for this, but don't force anything. At the same time, raise your arms. Gaze ahead.

Hold this position for as long as you can without breathing. Then slowly lower your chest to the floor again as you exhale. Rest your head to one side and relax. Do several rounds.

Benefits: In addition to being an excellent way to strengthen the lower back, serpent pose stretches and opens the chest. It alleviates respiratory ailments such as asthma. It is useful to promote good circulation and a healthy heart. It also encourages you to let go of any negative emotions you might be holding onto.

Yoga Poses for Looking Younger

Generally, any inverted positions will reverse the effects of gravity on your face, making you appear younger and holding off the onset of sagging facial features that make you look old. In particular, *surya namaskara* and inverted pose (above) are beneficial in this regard. Another pose good for maintaining a youthful appearance is *halasana*, the plough pose.

Halasana / Plough Pose

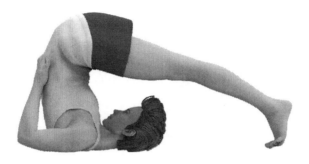

Lie flat on your back with your legs together and your arms by your sides, with the palms facing down. Inhale and lift your legs from the floor without bending them, letting your abs do the work. Hold the breath, and push against the floor with your arms and hands so that your buttocks and back are lifted, vertebra by vertebra, in a rolling motion towards your head. Lower your legs over your head until your toes touch the floor above your head. If you can't make it quite that far, don't force it.

You may either hold the pose by pressing the palms against the floor, or bend the elbows and bring the palms against the back so that they support you that way. Hold the pose for as long as you are comfortable and breathe deeply, allowing the muscles, particularly in your upper back and neck, to relax.

You may resume the original supine position by slowly lowering the back, vertebra by vertebra, to the floor, then the buttocks, then legs. If you have been holding your palms against your back, first return them face down to the floor, then lower your back, buttocks, and legs.

Another way of getting into plough pose is to start with inverted pose (above) or its more advanced version, *sarvangasana*, the shoulder stand pose.

Benefits: Plough pose has many benefits, including promoting a youthful appearance by allowing blood to flow to the face. It also strengthens the abdominal muscles and massages the organs of the abdomen, promoting good digestion. It stretches and strengthens the muscles in the back and neck, removing tension from the shoulders and neck and increasing blood flow to that part of the body. Plough pose, along with inverted pose, will also decrease acne.

Virabhadrasana I / Warrior Pose I

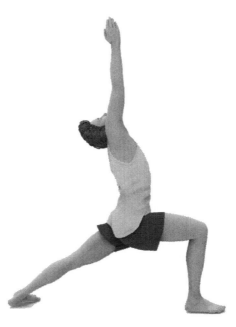

The warrior sequence of poses involves three poses, the third of which is more challenging. These poses are excellent for toning muscles in the legs, butt, core, back, and arms, as well as encouraging circulation and restoring a youthful appearance. They also instill a sense of youthful confidence and courage, making your awareness sharper and more focused—the attitudes of a determined warrior.

This sequence of three poses is named for a legendary warrior, Virabhadra. The first pose imitates his stance as, summoned by Shiva, he rose up from the earth with the swords in his hands piercing the sky.

Stand straight with your arms at your sides. Stretch your arms above your head, joining the palms. As you inhale, stretch your legs apart, so that they span about two thirds of your height.

Then exhale as you turn to face the left. At the same time, rotate your left foot so that it points in the same direction. Bend your left knee and lean in that direction, with your back arched and arms still pointing upwards and your eyes aimed at your hands about your head. Your right leg should be straight and stretched behind you.

Hold the position for a count of five, then straighten your left leg again. Rotate your left foot back to its original position. Then turn to the right, rotate the right foot, and repeat the pose on the right side.

Repeat for five to ten rounds. Then exhale and return to the standing position.

Benefits: Warrior pose I strengthens muscles in the legs, feet, back, shoulders, and arms. It also stretches the hips and calves. It increases balance. Warrior pose I also improves concentration.

Virabhadrasana II / Warrior Pose II

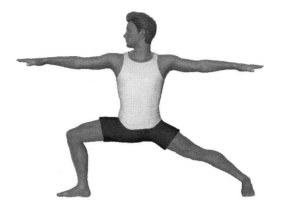

The second warrior pose imitates Virabhadra's stance as he spotted his enemy from afar.

From the same standing position as before, again stretch the legs apart to the same width as before. Stretch your arms to either side, parallel to the ground. Then, again rotate the left foot so that it points straight to the left. Lean into that direction with your left leg, bending the knee. Keep your back straight. Your gaze should move along the left arm. Hold the pose for a count of five.

Then return to the stretched, square stance. Repeat the same movements on the right side.

Repeat for five to ten rounds, then return to the original standing position.

Benefits: Warrior pose II tones the leg muscles, arms, and back. It improves balance. Cognitively, it instills a sense of courage.

Virabhadrasana III / Warrior Pose III

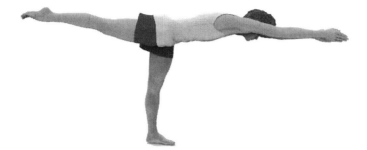

The third warrior pose imitates Virabhadra's stance as he thrust forward with his sword, slicing off the head of his enemy.

This one's a bit tricky and looks like something out of a kung fu flick. Once you're comfortable with the previous two warrior poses, you can perform the third Virabhadrasana.

Again begin standing straight, and again assume the squared stance with legs stretched apart. Turn your left leg so that it points to the left. Then, exhaling, lift your right foot off the ground at the same time as leaning to the left with your entire body, arms stretched all the way out.

The aim is to form a kind of T-shape, with all of your weight balanced on the left leg, the right leg stretched out behind you and your arms stretched out in front. That way your entire body is parallel to the ground.

Hold your balance for a count of five, if you can. If you can't keep it for that long, return to the squared stance—and try not to fall! (But if you do, no big deal. Just rinse and repeat.) Then repeat on the right side.

Benefits: Virabhadrasana III improves agility and balance. Just as it imitates an extremely focused sword thrust, this asana improves concentration and focus. It tones the muscles in the leg, as well as strengthening your core.

Yoga Poses for Relaxation

In this day and age, our lives are too busy and hectic, and we are so enthralled by technology that, even when we get some time to ourselves, we keep ourselves busy, feeding a constant stream of information into our heads. The result is that we rarely, if ever, take time to ourselves to show ourselves kindness by just *resting*. In fact, we may not even know how to rest.

Resting doesn't just mean sleeping or having a lie down, although it can mean that, too. Resting can also mean taking the time to do meditation, or eating your favorite food, or gardening—if that is the sort of thing you find pleasant and relaxing. Actually, anything that you do for intrinsic enjoyment and that leaves you feeling renewed and energetic can be called rest.

Relaxation is indispensable to any yoga practice. If you do not take the time to rest, you will suffer in body and mind. The poses in this chapter are aimed at producing a state of physical and mental relaxation.

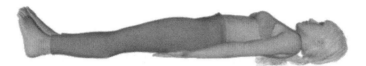

Lie on your back with your feet slightly apart and your arms a few inches away from either side of your body, palms up and fingers relaxed. Close your eyes and let your whole body and mind relax. If you like, you can focus your mind on the breath as described in the meditation chapter, allowing your mind to merge and identify with the breath. In this way, your body and mind reach a state of natural and deep relaxation.

You may stay in corpse pose for as long as you like. It typically comes at the end of a yoga session, but you can also lie down in *shavasana* any time you become physically or mentally tired and need to rest. Time and practice will increase your sensitivity to your own needs, so that you are well attuned to when you need to rest.

Benefits: Corpse pose provides profound relaxation for body and mind. This allows the muscle tissues to repair themselves and decreases stress and anxiety. It allows you to recover your energy, particularly after a vigorous practice session. It decreases blood pressure and calms compulsive over-thinking.

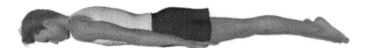

Lie flat on your stomach with your legs straight, the tops of your feet stretched along the floor. Your arms should be stretched forward with the palms facing downward. Place your forehead on the floor. Allow all the muscles in your body to relax completely, and breathe in a natural way, without forcing or changing anything about the breath. As in corpse pose, you may wish to practice mindfulness of the breath here, counting from one to ten, to induce deeper relaxation.

Keep this position for as long as you like, simply resting without any concern.

Benefits: Similarly to corpse pose, reversed corpse pose allows the body-mind complex to relax deeply. It also is useful for slipped disc, stiffness of the neck, and to correct bad posture.

Makarasana / Crocodile Pose

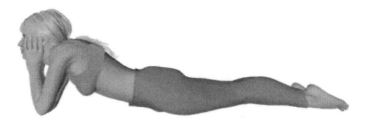

Lie flat on your stomach, as in reversed corpse pose, with your toes pointing out. Lift your head and chest from the floor, and bring your chin to rest in your palms, propping it up by your elbows. Allow your whole body and all your muscles to relax. Close your eyes and breathe naturally, without trying to alter the breath.

If there is too much strain on your neck, move your elbows apart to lower your head slightly. You should feel an equal pressure on your neck and lower back, so adjust your elbows to find the right balance. The posture should feel comfortable and relaxed without any strain. Remain in crocodile pose for as long as you like.

Benefits: As with corpse pose and reversed corpse pose, crocodile pose induces profound relaxation and decreases stress and anxiety. Like reversed corpse pose, it also improves such spinal disorders as slipped disc. Crocodile pose has one big advantage over the previous two poses: it makes it easier to breathe deeply from your belly, using your diaphragm to draw the breathe instead of your chest.

Contraindications: Don't do crocodile pose if it causes you to feel any pain in your back.

Salamba Bhujangasana / Sphinx Pose

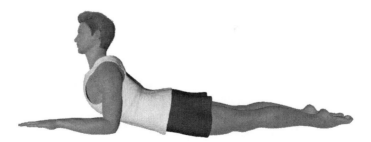

Lie on the floor on your stomach. Your toes should stretch downward. With your hands and belows touching the floor, breathe in and push with your arms, lifting your chest, head, and shoulders from the floor. Your navel should still be touching the floor. Your head should be held straight up, gazing forward like the sphinx. Breathe slowly and gently, holding the position for a count of ten. Then slowly lower yourself to the floor again.

Benefits: Sphinx pose strengthens the spine. It stretches the abdomen and the abdominal organs, stimulating digestion. It expands the chest and shoulders. This pose improves circulation and releases tension from stress.

Gomukhasana / Cow's Face Pose

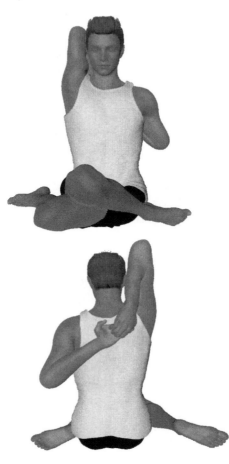

Sit with your legs flat on the ground and your back straight, hands resting on your thighs.

Bring your left foot under your right knee and place it on the outside of your right hip. Then bring the right foot over the left leg, and place your right foot outside your left hip. The knees should be one on top of the other.

Inhaling, stretch your left arm out to the side. Turn your palm first down, then facing backwards, so that your thumb points down. Exhaling, bring the arm behind your back and place it against your lower back. Then move the arm up your back as far as possible, keeping it to the left of the spine.

Inhale and stretch your right arm forward. Turn the palm upward, then raise the arm vertically. Exhale and bend it over your head and behind your back. Try to grasp the left fingers with the right, if you can.

Hold for a minute or two. Then unclasp your hands, return to the original position and repeat, switching right and left.

If your fingers can't reach each other, use a strap. Hang it over your shoulder, then grasp it with the lower hand. When the upper hand comes over the head and reaches down, it also grabs the strap. Then pull with the upper arm to stretch the lower one. Don't strain—the idea is to increase flexibility *gradually*.

Benefits: Cow's face pose stretches the legs, shoulders, neck, back, and arms. It opens the hips and reduces stiffness in the back, neck, and shoulders. Psychologically, it is an excellent way to relieve stress and anxiety. It restores energy when you're tired and improves your posture.

Dandasana / Staff Pose

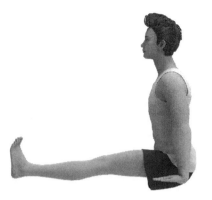

Sit on the floor with your legs out in front of you and together. Keep your back straight and vertical. Place your hands at your side, palms down on the floor.

If your hamstrings are tight, this might be uncomfortable. In that case, practice getting the position right by sitting with your back straight against a wall.

Benefits: Staff pose strengthens the muscles in your back, helps align your spine and sitting bones, and improves posture.

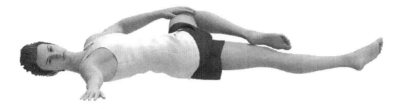

Lie on your back as in *shavasana*, with your arms at your sides. Bend your left leg, bringing the foot up against the side of your right knee. Grasp your left knee with your right hand, and pull it towards the ground.

Stretch your left arm to the left and rest it on the floor, palm up. Turn your face to the left as far as you can and gaze in that direction. Don't lift your shoulder blades from the floor.

Hold that for a minute and relax into it. Then repeat on the other side.

Benefits: The reclining twist improves flexibility in the spine. It stimulates the abdominal organs. It relaxes and widens the shoulders and hips. It eases stress and anxiety. It also improves digestion.

Garudasana / Eagle Pose (seated)

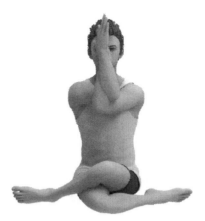

Begin in a seated position. Bend your right leg and bring it under your left knee, and place the foot outside your left hip. Then bring the right foot outside the left hip. The left knee should be resting on top of the right knee.

Then stretch your arms out in front of you. Keeping your arms straight, cross your right arm over your left a bit above the elbows. Bend your left elbow while keeping your right arm straight. Your left palm should face to the right.

Then bend your right arm, with the palm facing to the left. Press the right palm with the fingers of the left hand. If you can't do that, then use the left fingers to grasp the right thumb. Lift your elbows so that your upper arms are at a right angle to your body. Your forearms should also be vertical, so that your elbows also form a right angle. Hold that position for a count of ten to twenty breaths, breathing deeply into the area between your shoulder blades.

Benefits: This pose is second to none for relaxing muscle tension in hard-to-reach areas of the upper back and neck. You will probably feel it right away reaching long-neglected muscles that needed some tender loving care. If you want to give a little extra stretch, lift your elbows slightly.

There is a more advanced, standing version of this pose that requires excellent balance and focus to pull off. But I've presented the simpler version here as an introduction, so you can get the benefits of this position right away.

Yoga for Reproductive Health

The poses in this section encourage reproductive health in men and women, improve sexual function, and balance the sex drive.

Vajrasana / Diamond Pose

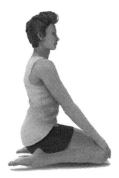

Kneel down with the feet tucked under your buttocks. The big toes should touch each other, while the heels point outward, pressed beneath the hips. Rest your palms on your thighs or knees, keeping your back straight. With your eyes closed, relax your body and mind. Rest with mindfulness of the inhalation and exhalation of the breath. You can sit like this for a long time in meditation.

If you find that the pressure on your heels hurts your feet, try placing a pillow between your butt and your heels.

Benefits: Vajrasana improves digestion and can be practiced after meals. It relieves common stomach discomfort.

It strengthens the pelvis and alleviates excessive libido. It relieves menstrual pain in women and encourages a regular cycle.

Virasana / Hero's Pose

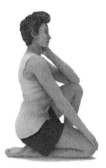

Start in vajrasana or diamond pose. Raise the left knee and place the left foot flat on the ground, next to the right knee. Rest your upper arm or left elbow on the raised knee, and rest your chin in the palm of your left hand. Keep your spine straight. You may just rest naturally in this position for as long as you like.

Then, return to vajrasana and switch sides. Rest again.

Benefits: Hero's pose tones and optimizes the organs of the abdomen. It also improves reproductive function. This pose also increases focus and encourages clear thinking. It reduces excessive, worrisome, or negative thoughts and relaxes the mind, making it very clear and precise.

Ardha Titali Asana / Half Butterfly Pose

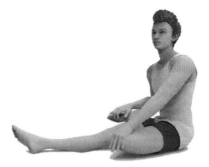

Sit on the floor with your legs straight in front of you. Pull your left foot in and rest it on top of your right thigh, bring it all the way in so it touches your waste.

Hold the left toe with the right hand. Your left hand should grab your left knee. Your back and neck should be straight, while the right leg is still stretched out straight in front of you.

With each inbreath, pull the left knee up towards your chest without straining. Then, as you breathe out, push the knee all the way to the floor. Repeat this motion 20 times.

Return to the starting position, then do it again with your right leg this time.

Benefits: This helps open up the hips and make the knees flexible. It prepares the body for sitting long sessions of meditation. It also balances the reproductive function.

Purna Titali Asana / Full Butterfly Pose

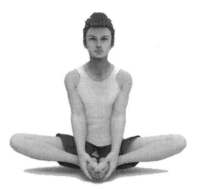

As before, sit with your back straight and legs stretched out in front of you. Pull both the feet in as far as you can, bringing the heels close to the groin. The soles of your feet should touch. Grasp your knees with your hands and relax the thighs.

Try to keep your back straight throughout this pose. Bring your knees up and down in a bouncing motion, pushing down on your knees with your hands on the downward movement. Try to push them all the way to the ground, but don't strain.

Do about 50 of these movements, then return to the original position.

Benefits: The same as half butterfly pose, but more so. It also relieves tiredness and ache in the legs and knees.

Shashankasana / Hare's Pose

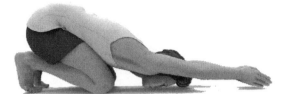

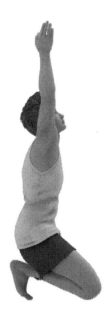

Start in vajrasana. Then, while inhaling, swivel both arms and point them straight up above the head, keeping them shoulders-width apart. Exhale and bend forward from the waist, bringing your arms and forehead all the way to the floor. Keep your buttocks touching your heels as much as you can. Hold that position for a count of ten, relaxing fully.

Then raise your arms and body all the way up again. Finally, slowly lower your arms to the original position. Repeat four times.

Benefits: Hare's pose stretches the spine, pulling the vertebrae away from each other and allowing them to realign. The up and down pivot from the hip strengthens the muscles in the pelvis. It remedies reproductive disorders in both men and women and encourages optimal sexual functioning.

Yoga Poses for Meditation

Sukhasana / Comfortable Position

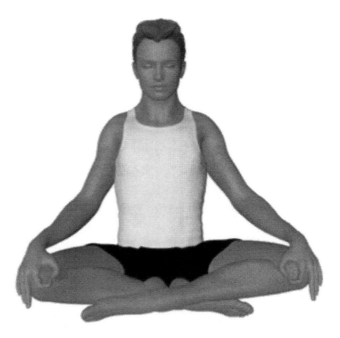

The easiest meditation position by far for beginners is *sukhasana* or the "comfortable pose." In this position, you cross your legs as you normally would when sitting on the floor. The spine and neck should be straight but relaxed, without any strain. Because of the position of the legs, this can be a little hard to achieve in *sukhasana*, so it will be much easier to keep your back straight if your butt is seated on a cushion two or three inches off the ground. Otherwise, if you can manage it, your back will feel more comfortable, and you will be able to keep your spine straight for longer periods of time, if you can sit in some of the more advanced meditation postures, such as the lotus position.

Your hands should rest in a *mudra* in which the forefinger rests on the inside of the thumb, forming a circle, and the other three fingers are extended but relaxed. The palms may face either up or down, resting on the knees, with the arms stretched forward and the elbows slightly bent.

Tilt your head slightly forward. You may keep your eyes either open or closed. If you hold your eyes open, allow them to rest on a point about four to five feet in front of you in empty space, your gaze relaxed and defocused.

Benefits:The main benefit of *sukhasana* is that it is easy to maintain for people whose bodies are unable to sit in the more difficult meditation positions. Otherwise, for longer periods of meditation, one of the other postures that allows the knees to touch the floor will yield much greater stability.

Padmasana / Lotus Position

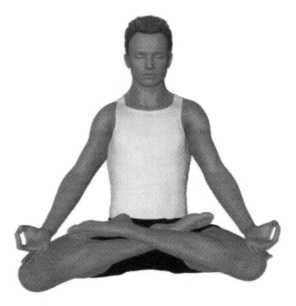

The *lotus position* is the classic and most famous meditation pose. If you can manage it, great. If you can't, don't sweat it. With *padmasana*, as with other yoga positions, it's very important not to force your body to do anything it doesn't want to do, or else you risk injuring yourself. So if you can't get yourself into the right position, simply practice the more dynamic poses from the health chapter and your flexibility will increase. In time, *padmasana* will be within reach for you. For now, if lotus position is just too much, try less demanding positions such as *sukhasana* and half-lotus.

This posture is famously hard to achieve for beginners and can cause pain on the legs, but if you are going to sit in meditation for long periods of time, it allows the highest level of stability and ease on the back. Moreover, the posture is especially good at allowing the body's *prana*, or subtle energy, to flow in a way that lends itself to deep and powerful meditative awareness.

To sit in the lotus position, sit cross-legged on the mat or cushion, with your left foot resting on the right thigh, and right foot resting on the left thigh. The back should be held straight but relaxed, with minimal effort and without tension, as if the spine were a stack of coins. The knees should touch the ground. The shoulders should be held somewhat back, like a vulture's wings, and the tongue rest at the roof of the mouth. The *mudra* or gesture of the hands may vary, but usually the hands rest, palms up, on the knees, with the nail of the forefinger touching the inside of the thumb.

Benefits: The lotus position allows for stability during long periods of sitting meditation. The posture not only allows a steady, sitting position without movement, it also encourages the mind to naturally calm down and rest in meditative awareness. Physically, this pose strengthens posture and spinal alignment, as well as improving digestion by allowing blood to flow to the digestive tract.

Contraindications: Do not attempt this posture if you have weak or injured knees. Also avoid it if you have great difficulty achieving it, or if sitting in *padmasana* causes physical pain. Before you attempt *padmasana*, it is good to practice other yoga positions that loosen the muscles and increase flexibility. If you suffer from sciatica, you should also avoid the lotus position.

Variations: In the variation called *ardha-padmasana* or half-lotus, one leg is drawn in and rests on the floor against the inside of the opposite thigh, while the other leg rests on top of the other thigh. This position is easier and requires less flexibility in the legs than the full lotus position.

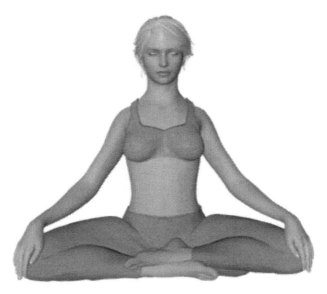

The right foot rests against the inside of the left thigh with the heel pressing against the perineum, so that this area is sitting on top of the right heel. Then the left leg is drawn in, with the left ankle resting on the right ankle. Tuck the toes of the left foot between the calf and thigh of the right leg. In the final position, the left feel should press into the pubic area above the genitals, so that the genitals are between the left and right heels.

There are two versions of this pose, one for women and one for men. The version for women is called *siddha yoni asana* and is much the same as described above, but with left and right reversed, with the *left* heel pressing against the labia, and the right foot on top, its heel pressing against the clitoris.

The hands and the rest of the body are held as in *sukhasana* and lotus position, described above.

Benefits:*Siddhasana* may allow for similar stability to the lotus position for those who aren't flexible enough to sit in full lotus. It benefits people who suffer from high blood pressure and prostate problems. It redirects the body's subtle energy upwards, away from the genitals. That means it decreases the sexual libido. I'll leave it up to you to decide whether or not that's a benefit!

Sequences

The individual poses are all well and good, but how should you use them as part of a coherent practice, and in what order? It's important to have a sequence for practicing the asanas. It gives structure to your yoga practice and helps you focus.

A Basic Yoga Sequence

This is a basic, all-purpose yoga sequence that you can use as a daily practice:

1. Begin by sitting in a meditation pose such as *sukhasana*. Take some time to center yourself through mindfulness meditation or rhythmic breathing (described in the chapter on Breathing).

2. Stand up, then lean forward and perform downward-facing dog.

3. Next, perform the *Surya Namaskar* series several times – at least three. You may do it slowly or quickly, according to your preference.

4. Do v*rkasana*, tree pose, for a couple of minutes on each leg, or as long as you can maintain your balance.

5. Lower your feet to the ground, then move into *trikonasana,* triangle pose. Perform this pose on both sides.

6. Next, perform *uttitha parsvakonasana,* or extended side-angle pose, on both sides.

7. Return to a standing position, then sit on the floor in *dandasana,* staff pose.

8. From the upright position, lean forward into *paschimottanasana,* or a forward bend.

9. Return to *dandasana,* then draw your ankles in toward your groin and do *purna titali asana,* the full butterfly pose. If that's too difficult, perform half butterfly pose with each leg.

10. Again sit in *dandasana,* then stretch your legs apart and lean forward to in *upavistha konasana,* wide angle pose.

11. Return to *dandasana,* then perform *naukasana,* boat pose.

12. Lie face down and perform *sarpasana,* snake pose.

13. Move onto your back and arch your back upwards in *setu asana,* bridge pose.

14. Lower your back to the ground again, then assume inverted pose, *vipareeta karani asana.*

15. Resume lying down. Then do *jathari parivartaranasana* or reclining twist.

16. Finally just lie on your back in corpse pose, *shavasana.* Just let your mind and body relax completely for as long as you like. You may find that your mind is in a naturally meditative state. That's because loosening tension in your muscles and stretching various parts of your body stimulates prana, or subtle energy, to move through your system, which acts as a support for balanced, meditative awareness.

You don't have to follow this sequence exactly, but it gives you a good sense of how a yoga sequence is structured.

It starts with meditation and Surya Namaskara. Then comes a group of standing poses. Next you perform sitting poses. Finally, there is a group of poses that are performed either lying down, or starting from a lying position, ending with corpse pose.

So the structure is standing – sitting – lying down. You can add or subtract any poses to this sequence as appropriate. For example, if you want to give a little extra love to your spine, you can do *ardha matsyendrasana* with the other sitting poses—after *paschimottanasana*, say. Or if you find *upavistha konasana* to be too strenuous, you can just replace it with something more comfortable for your body. The asanas described in the beginning of this book are a good repository of beginner and intermediate yoga poses to draw on.

* * *

You might also prefer to do a sequence for a more specific purpose. The following is an example.

Sequence for Shoulders and Stress Relief

Stress is a ubiquitous ailment in modern life, and it often manifests physically, especially as pain and tension in the shoulders and upper back. A stiff neck and stiff shoulders, or poor posture with slouched shoulders, are very common problems. It doesn't help that many of us sit at a desk all day, bent over a screen, tapping and clicking away with no time to pay attention to our posture. This sequence is kind of a corrective to all these problems and will relieve stress and pain in the shoulders.

1. Begin with *surya namaskara*.

2. Standing up, perform downward-facing dog. Hold that for two minutes.

3. Then lower the body and hold it in plank pose, *phalakasana*, for two minutes.

4. Again do downward-facing dog, and again plank pose.

5. Stand up and perform *tadasana*, palm tree pose.

6. From there, do *trikonasana*.

7. Lower yourself to a seated position, move into *gomukhasana*, the cow faced pose. Perform on each side, giving a good stretch to each arm.

8. Then do *garudasana*, eagle pose, in the same way.

9. Lean forward into *paschimottanasana*, forward bending pose. Really let your back muscles relax as you pull with your hands.

10. Return to an upright position, then do *ardha matsyendrasana*, half spinal twist.

11. Lie down on your back and do *setu asana*, bridge pose.

12. Relax into *shavasana* for a moment.

13. Then lift your legs up into inverted pose, *vipareeta karani asana*.

14. From inverted pose, if you can manage it, bring your legs over your head and back down in *halasana*, plough pose.

Slowly return to a lying position, vertebra by vertebra, and finally rest in *shavasana*. Allow your body and mind to relax fully, and just breath deeply, sinking into a deep and restful state.

Breathing

The benefits of yoga are many, but you have to experience them for yourself before you begin to understand how yoga can have a profound effect on your life. It will improve your performance in many areas, including your professional and social lives, your emotional wellbeing, health, and sense of peace.

One of the things you will notice as you get further into practicing yoga is that you start paying attention to these other areas more closely. Yoga works best in harmony with other healthy practices, as part of a holistic approach to overall wellness. It works synergistically to bring the mind and body together as a working whole with coherence.

Coherence is something neuroscientist and performance expert Alan Watkins talks about extensively in his book, *Coherence: The Secret Science of Brilliant Leadership*. What coherence means is that the functions of body and mind are working rhythmically and harmoniously, instead of fluctuating chaotically between different states.

When your physiology—for example, your heart rate—becomes chaotic, the frontal lobe of your brain shuts down. The frontal lobe is responsible for higher-order thinking, logic, and decision making. Anything that requires concentration and problem solving draws on the brain power of the frontal lobe. And to be effective in navigating the twists and turns of our lives and jobs, we really need that brain power at our disposal. That's why it's critical to bring the chaotic fluctuations of body and mind down to a minimum and increase coherence as much as possible.

Our brain's toolkit for dealing with the many problems of life was put together to deal with pretty primitive situations, when our ancestors lived on the savanna and were mostly concerned with basic concerns like food, shelter, and avoiding dangerous predators. So in many ways we're poorly equipped to deal with the challenges of life. Fortunately, however, there are some performance hacks we can use to make our creaky, ancient system work better for the demands of modern life. When mind and body are working together optimally, it's truly amazing how much more effective you can become.

One of the best ways to establish coherence or stability of body and mind is through working with the breath. According to Watkins, there are twelve aspects of the breath that we can train ourselves to control, but he believes only the first three of them are essential for improving coherence. Still, I'll mention all twelve of them here, because some of them are important for *pranayama*, the branch of yoga that deals with breath control.

- Rhythm – a steady ratio of inbreath to outbreath
- Smoothness – the evenness of the breath
- Location of attention – where on your body is your mind focused as you control your breath?
- Speed
- Pattern – a specific ratio of inbreath to outbreath
- Volume – how much air you take in with one breath
- Depth – how deeply the air enters the lungs
- Entrainment – synchronization of systems in the body, mostly unconscious
- Resistance – any obstruction or constriction of airflow, for example, by constricting the nostrils
- Mechanics – use of muscles such as the diaphragm
- Flow patterns – of air through the body
- Special techniques – such as meditation techniques

The idea of rhythmic breathing is to work with the first three aspects. So you can breathe in for a count of 4, breathe out for a count of 6, and hold your breathe for a count of 2. Or you can do 5:5, or 3:6, or any variation that feels more comfortable to you. For this practice, the precise number is not nearly as important as the consistency of the rhythm. The rhythm itself brings your body's rhythms into coherence, which in turn stabilizes your feelings, emotions, and thoughts.

When you're breathing, make sure your breaths are *smooth* from beginning to end. Taking rough, jagged, or uneven breaths is going to increase variance and decrease coherence. That's the second aspect of the exercise.

Finally, you want to focus your attention in the central area of your chest, near the heart or heart chakra. That will bring your awareness deeper into the body, making you feel more centered. Because this area is also connected to positive emotion, it will encourage an overall feeling of psychological wellbeing. Just feel the rise and fall of your chest, and focus on the feeling of the breath passing through this central area.

This kind of breathing is also good practice for performing the asanas of yoga. When you are doing asanas, your breath should be rhythmic and smooth, and your awareness should be on different areas of your body.

Pranayama

As already mentioned, the tradition of yoga has its own body of practices for working with the breath. These are part of the science of pranayama. I deal with the subject more extensively in my books about chakras and kundalini. Here I'll just give a basic introduction to the idea so you can get your feet wet.

According to pranayama, the breath is connected with *prana*, a subtle energy that animates the body and the world. Or, if you prefer, you could think of it as an energy that runs through your subjective experience of your own body and the world. It doesn't really matter. The point is that the practices working with prana can enhance your body and mind greatly.

In your own subtle body, prana courses through a system of energy channels. There are many such channels, but the main ones are three and run from your root chakra near the anus up to the crown cakra of your head:

- *Ida* is on the left side of the body and has a feminine, passive quality.
- *Pingala* is on the right side of the body and its quality is masculine and active.
- *Sushumna* runs through the center and is neither masculine nor femine, passive nor active—its energy is nondual.

The ultimate goal of pranayama is to cause the subtle energies to enter the central sushumna channel and rise to the crown of the head. But be warned: this can be extremely dangerous without preparation and the guidance of a qualified spiritual master.

The subtle body is like a map of all the aspects and levels of your being. As human beings, we are animals, but we are also something more than our biology. We are also capable of achieving great intellectual and spiritual heights. So the chakras are arranged all the way from the lowest level, which has to do with the simplest biological functions, to the crown chakra, which is level of highest spiritual attainment and knowledge of absolute consciousness.

None of us is *just* a physical being or *just* a spiritual being. The lesson of Indian spirituality is that we are rooted in the material, biological level of life as well as the higher divine plane. We always have to keep our feet on the ground, to touch the basic solidity of existence. There is no escaping it: if we try to soar up and away from our earthly life, like Icarus, we will come plummeting back down to the earth.

At the same time, earthiness is not the totality our being. We are composed even more of sky. Modern physics tells us that, despite the appearance of solidity, the atoms of our body are quite spread out. It's very roomy in here. We are 99.9999999999996% empty space.

So heaven and earth meet together in one being: the human. Yoga develops the physical aspect of our being as a basis for working with the spiritual aspect. If we focus on the one and neglect the other, we are like a bird trying to fly with only one wing.

Sushumna is like a cosmic axis that connects earth and sky. It allows communication to take place between matter and spirit. But before that can happen, the body has to be developed so that it's not blown away by the raw power of our innermost spiritual being.

Nadi shodhana / Alternate Nostril Breathing

As suggested by *ida* and *pingala,* yoga teaches that our being has both masculine and feminine sides to it. That's not some sexist ideology: each of us has both within us, and we tend to prefer one mode over the other. These also have to do with the left and right brains. The left brain controls the right half of the body, which is the domain of *pingala,* the masculine. The right brain controls the left half of the body, which contains *ida,* the left or feminine channel.

Men tend to prefer masculine energy—but *not all men.* Women likewise *tend* to prefer feminine energy, but of course many women are exceptional. And no woman relies on feminine energy *all* the time. We are complex beings with many sides.

Relying too much on either energy can be a problem. Too much masculine energy can make you over-aggressive, overanalytic, and left-brained. As the saying goes, when your only tool is a hammer, everything is a nail. You just try to bulldoze your way through life—a crude and apish approach.

Too much feminine energy, and you become too meek and passive, too emotional and right-brained. Then it's easy for others to take advantage of you.

Yoga always seeks balance between opposing forces. That's why all the asanas above require equal time for both left and right sides of the body. The fact is that we have both masculine and feminine energy at our disposal, so why not make the best use of what we have? That way we have balance in our lives and can always find an appropriate way to do things. It's much better than being lopsided all the time.

Nadi shodhana, or alternate nostril breathing, balances the masculine and feminine aspects of our being by controlling the way prana flows through ida and pingala. Through this practice, you give equal time to ida and pingala and find the happy center.

1. For this practice, choose one of the seated meditation postures such as lotus position, or the pose of the masters. Lotus position is best, because of the way the feet press against the subtle channels in the legs. But choose whichever position is comfortable. Don't strain yourself!

2. Spend a few minutes just relaxing and performing the rhythmic breathing described earlier. This brings your physiological rhythms into coherence and calms the mind.

3. Leave your left hand resting on your knee, and press your right index and middle fingers between your eyebrows, at the third-eye chakra. This stimulates insight and awareness.

4. Breathe out completely. Then press your right thumb against the right side of your nose. Inhale through your left nostril to a fixed count of 5 seconds.

(You can vary this number according to your comfort level, but keep it consistent throughout the practice!)

5. Open your right nostril, then close the left nostril by pressing your ring and pinky fingers sgainst the side of your nose. Breathe out through the right nostril, again for 5 seconds.

(If you prefer a different length of time, make sure the length of inbreath and outbreath is equal.)

6. Again breathe in through the right nostril as before. Repeat this ten times.

7. Perform the alternate nostril breathing again, this time inhaling through your right nostril and exhaling through your left nostril. Just as before, but with the opposite nostrils. Repeat ten times.

As you breathe in and out, let your mind follow the breath. Just let your awareness melt into the breath, becoming one with it. You can perform this cycle as many times as you like. It's good to do it in the early morning or early evening. You can also do it any time you feel stressed or overwhelmed and just need to find your center again. It immediately introduces balance by equalizing the energy between the masculine and feminine polarities of your body and mind.

Afterwards, you may prefer to just sit in quiet meditation for any length of time. Nadi shodhana is an excellent way to calm and prepare the mind for less complex forms of meditation, and you may find that it allows you to go deeper into relaxed but alert concentration.

Jala Neti

By now you've probably figured out that breathing is very important in yoga, especially breathing connected with the nose and the nostrils. So it's important to keep the nasal passages very clean. Mucus can always build up because of illness or allergies, too much pollution, and so on.

Jala neti cleans it all up and allows air to flow easily through the nose. The practice might seem kind of weird at first, but I guarantee you it makes you feel 100% better. So don't let it freak you out. Especially if you're having difficulty breathing or suffering from any congestion, performing jala neti will wash out all the mucus and pollution from your nasal passages. This allows you to perform yoga and pranayama much more comfortably.

Jala neti involves pouring a saline solution through one nostril so that it flows out of the other nostril, taking built up mucus, dust, and toxic pollution with it. That sounds awful, but it's not. It's perfectly comfortable and is probably the most effective treatment for congestion from colds, allergies, and sinusitis. So give it a try. It's probably the least bizarre of the six *shatkarmas* or purifying practices—believe it or not.

How to do it

To do jala neti, you need a special kind of pot called a neti pot. It's open at the top and has a long spout with a tip that will fit comfortably inside your nostril. A pot that contains about 500 ml of water does best. You can easily order a neti pot online. Your local drug store might also carry them.

Mix warm water, of approximate body temperature, and salt. Don't use iodized salt or salt with additives such as anti-caking agents. Pure sea salt or kosher salt do very nicely.

There mix should be one teaspoon of salt for every 500 ml of water. Stir well, so the salt is completely dissolved.

Then pour a small amount of water from the spout. This removes any water from the spout that didn't get the proper mix of salt to water.

Then, leaning over a sink and tilting your head slightly, put the tip of the spout in your left nostril and tilt the pot. Pouring the solution into your left nostril until the water comes out of the right. Keep pouring until the pot is empty. While you're doing this, continue to breathe through your mouth.

The water should come straight out of your nostril and not run down your chin, so adjust your position accordingly.

When the pot is empty, blow your nose gently over the sink to expel any mucus or extra water that remain inside. Then refill the pot and repeat with the other side.

Afterwards, you can lean forward in a bathtub or shower, with your hands on your knees. Move your head to the left and the right, allowing excess water to drain from your eyes. Breathe vigorously through your nose to dry it out.

A more advanced technique involves sucking the solution through the nostril and spitting it out from the mouth. But I would recommend mastering the first technique before you try the advanced version.

Benefits: Jala neti is obviously useful for clearing up congestion. But it also removes obstructions to airflow in the left and right nostrils. This makes it easier to practice pranayama. It also balances the prana in the left and right channels, which balances activity between the two hemispheres of the brain as well as the energy in the body. It stabilizes your mind, calms your mood and alleviates stress.

How to Meditate

So now that we've gone over the different meditation positions, it will probably be useful if we actually talk a bit about *how* to meditate. Meditation is all the rage these days, with a lot of scientific research to back up its many benefits. It is not just used in therapy, but also in offices and at home to improve people's overall quality of life.

Meditation is proven to lower stress, increase concentration and cognitive performance, reduce anxiety and depression, and elevate your mood. The good news is, it's also easy to do, so if you have any doubt or hesitation about your ability to get into the practice, don't worry. Just try it out for five minutes.

Sit in one of the meditation positions described above, with your back straight but in a relaxed posture. You'll probably find that sitting on a cushion helps to decrease strain on your back and allow you to sit still for longer periods of time.

Your eyes may be open or closed. It's up to you. If you open your eyes, keep your gaze several feet in front of you and pointing downward, either resting on a point in space or on the floor. Either way, allow the eyes to relax, without any strain or strong focus.

Take a moment to feel the mass and weight of your body where you're sitting. Feel the pressure of your body pressing onto the floor or cushion, the weight of your feet or knees on the floor. Allow yourself to get a real sense of your body's weight where it comes into contact with the ground.

Then, take a couple of deep, heavy breaths—basically like sighing. This helps release any tension you're holding in your body. With your attention, scan the different parts of your body, trying to notice any tension or pain, or alternately any pleasurable sensation. You don't have to try to do anything with the tension, particularly, or try to change it. Just notice and acknowledge that it's there.

Now direct your attention to your breathing, to the in-and-out movements of your breath. Try to really feel the breath—the cold on your nostrils as you breathe in, the feeling of your lungs expanding, the diaphragm opening up. Feel the heat in your nose as you exhale, and the falling sensation of your chest as the breath leaves your body.

Don't try to concentrate in a tense way, but just allow the mind to rest on its object. The mind should melt into the breath and identify with it, in a relaxed way.

In the beginning, it helps to count the breath. So with each breath, count, *one, two, three*, etc., all the way up to *ten*. Then, start over again from *one*. If your mind wanders or you get distracted by thoughts or emotions, don't worry about it. Just gently return your mind to the breath, and gently resume counting again from one.

That's it! Sit like that, with your attention resting on the breath, for five to ten minutes. If you find yourself checking the time again and again, use an app on your phone to give you a chime when it's time to finish up your session, so that you can take your mind off the ticking of the clock.

Maintaining a consistent, daily meditation practice does wonders for your stress level and mood, giving you a happier, fuller experience of life. Just a short, five-minute meditation session in the morning sets the right mood for the rest of the day. Combined with the other yoga positions discussed in this book, meditation is a powerful way of increasing your overall wellbeing and quality of life.

If you would like to know more about meditation, I invite you to check out The Meditation Beginner's Bible on Amazon.

http://a.co/bSeob16

The Benefits of Yoga

Over the past decade or so, a vast amount of scientific research has been carried out to investigate the benefits of Yoga for the human mind and body. The National Institute of Health has spent millions of dollars toward research on yoga, and nowadays it seems like new studies claiming new benefits of yoga are emerging every single day.

Thousands of peer-reviewed studies now been conducted on the benefits of yoga and the truth is practicing yoga has so many benefits that I could not possibly list them all in this book. So here are a few noteworthy benefits of developing a consistent yoga practice:

- Improves flexibility
- Builds muscle strength
- Reduces risk of heart disease and stroke
- Eases Asthma
- Improves memory
- Reduces insomnia
- Relieves pain more effectively than medication
- Perfects posture
- Lowers blood sugar
- Prevents cartilage and joint breakdown
- Protects spine
- Helps with weight loss
- Slows down the aging process
- Helps recover from addiction
- Helps beat depression
- Increases energy levels
- Increases endurance
- Enhances fertility

- Reduces pain associated with arthritis, fibromyaligia and other chronic conditions
- Boosts immune system functionality
- Increases blood flow
- Reduces stress and anxiety
- Improves relationships
- Improves athletic performance
- Lowers blood pressure more effectively than medication
- Regulates adrenal glands
- Improves focus
- Cultivates mental strength
- Fosters creativity
- Helps sleep deeper
- Decreases muscle tension
- Improves balance
- Enhances feelings of happiness and vitality
- Enhances self-awarenes
- Fosters peace of mind, happiness and joy
- Develops intuition
- Builds wisdom

Turning Yoga into a habit

Yoga is very much like going to the gym. Practice it regularly, and you become fit. Slack off, on the other hand, and you become chubby. In order to attain profound levels of inner peace, mental clarity, and happiness, you must practice yoga consistently.

In 2010, a study conducted at University College London showed that it takes on average 66 days to build a new habit. This means you need to invest about two months of effort before the behavior of meditation becomes automatic – something that you do without even thinking about it – a habit.

The key to making yoga automatic is to make it your top priority for the next 66 days. Yoga essentially has to become the most important activity in your day. Here are 9 ways to turn yoga into a habit:

Work on Your WHY

It's important to get crystal clear on why you want to make yoga a habit. Go through the list of benefits of yoga again and decide exactly why you want to practice yoga. Are you motivated to relieve stress, crush anxiety, be more successful or build stronger relationships? Make sure your WHY resonates deeply within you. When you have figured out your WHY, start visualizing your success. Imagine how your life will be when you achieve your goal and use this image as fuel and motivation to keep you going throughout your yoga journey.

Commit to the activity

Take a moment and make an oath to yourself to start doing yoga every single day from now on. Firmly set your intention that you are going to do this and never give up. Feel the energy rising inside your body and seal the commitment with your heart.

Start Small

There is no "right" amount of time to do yoga for. If you're a beginner, don't fall into the trap of trying to do yoga for hours on end. Your simply aren't trained to sustain it yet. You can start with as little as 5 minutes of daily yoga and you can gradually build your way up from there. The key is to not overwhelm yourself when you're starting out– 5 minutes of yoga everyday is much better than 5 hours of punctual yoga.

Decide on a fixed time and a trigger

When you are trying to develop a new habit, it's very important to have a trigger that reminds you to perform the new behavior around the same time everyday. The easiest way is to incorporate your meditation into your morning routine or evening routine. The key is to choose a trigger that makes it easy to juxtapose the new behavior onto an already existing habit. You can decide for example that you are going to meditate everyday day right after you brush your teeth in the morning or right before you go to bed.

Track Your Progress

Use a calendar to track your progress and make it visible. Mark down every time you follow through on your new habit. This will inspire you to keep going even when things get difficult. It will suddenly become more painful to break your streak. You can also use habit-tracking apps, which I have found to be extremely useful.

Be Accountable

Find an accountability buddy, preferably someone who is also looking to develop a long-term meditation practice. This will greatly increase your chances of success. When you have someone that holds you accountable, you will find it much more difficult to miss a session.

Split your sessions

One simple trick you can utilize to make your meditation more enjoyable is to split your meditation into two smaller sessions. This will allow you to easily increase your overall session length. Instead of trying to sit for a whole 30 minutes for example, it is much easier sit for 15 minutes in the morning and 15 minutes in the evening.

Reward Yourself

Whatever gets rewarded gets repeated. Your brain is constantly associating pain and pleasure to everything you do. So if you want your meditation habit to stick, trick your brain by rewarding yourself right after you have completed your meditation. It can be something as simple as giving yourself a pat on the back and saying to yourself: " Good job, you made progress today!".

Remember, consistent action is the only way to make mediation a habit. By practicing it everyday, you will create new neural pathways that will make the behavior automatic and you soon enough you won't even have to expand any willpower to sit down and meditate. Make meditation a long-term habit and it will transform every aspect of your life.

Conclusion

I hope this book was able to help you understand how practicing yoga can bring peace, happiness and joy into your life. The next step is to apply what you have learned and develop a long-term yoga practice. It can be a challenging process but I assure you that it is well worth it - You will enjoy a happier, more peaceful and balanced life free from stress, anxiety, and depression.

I wish you success on your yoga journey and I hope you quickly start reaping the amazing benefits that yoga has to offer.

Finally, if you enjoyed this book, then I'd like to ask you a favor. Would you be kind enough to share your thoughts and post a review of this book on Amazon?

Your voice is important for this book to reach as many people as possible. The more reviews this book gets, the more people will be able to find it and enjoy the incredible benefits of yoga.

Bonus: Free Guided Meditation Series (5 Audiobooks)

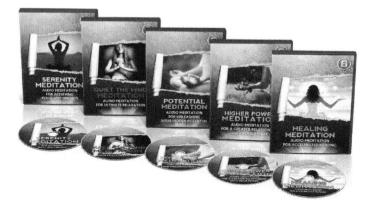

→ Go to http://freeguidedmeditationdownload.gr8.com to get your FREE Guided Meditation Series

You will get immediate access to:

- Healing Audio Meditation
- Higher Power Audio Meditation
- Potential Audio Meditation
- Quiet the Mind Audio Meditation
- Serenity Audio Meditation

You will also join my private kindle club and be the first to know about my upcoming kindle books!

Preview of
The Meditation Beginner's Bible

→ Available on Amazon

Introduction

From the outside meditation can seem like an esoteric, mystical endeavor exclusively reserved to enlightened monks and spiritual adepts. This could not be further from the truth. Meditation is not only accessible to anyone, it is extremely easy to learn and the benefits are only a few minutes away. In fact, a study by Dr Fadel Zeidan at Wake Forest Medical Center has shown only 80 minutes of meditation to be more effective for pain relief than even morphine.

In this book you will learn exactly why many highly successful people like Russell Simons, Arianna Huffington, Oprah Winfrey and Hugh Jackman set aside time off their busy schedules to engage in the life-changing practice of meditation.

Meditation can seem a bit daunting at first, especially if, like most of us, you're always up in your head, constantly dwelling on the past and worrying about the future. However, the moment you recognize that meditation is not about trying to empty your mind, but rather about observing your thoughts as they come and go without energizing them, you begin to awaken and meditation becomes the most blissful, transformative moment of the day.

This book will show you how to instill simple meditation techniques into your daily routine, inevitably leading you to a more successful, happier and healthier life.

Chapter 1 - What is meditation?

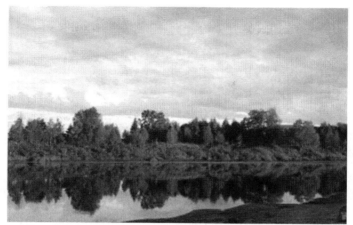

"The gift of learning to meditate is the greatest gift you can give yourself in this lifetime."
Sogyal Rinpoche

The word meditation and the word medicine come from the same Latin root "medicus" which means to cure. In the same way medicine cures sickness that exists inside the physical body by restoring it to a healthy state, meditation cures sickness that exists within the mind by returning it to its natural state of peace, joy and happiness.

But how does the mind become sick? Well, in our modern society most of us suffer from what we call compulsive thinking. We have this inner voice that is constantly thinking, ruminating the past, worrying about the future, and hence we never fully experience the present moment.

Take a few seconds right now and become aware of your breathing. Observe the changing sensations of your breath as you inhale and then exhale. Be aware of your lungs filling and emptying themselves. Become one with your breath and notice the subtle gap between your incoming and outcoming breath - let yourself completely dissolve into the activity of breathing.

If you did this little exercise, I bet you noticed your mind becoming a bit more still. When you rest your attention on your breath, you effectively step away from the chaotic impulses of the mind and you connect to your true Self – that eternal part of you that is beyond the ephemeral, ever-wavering physical realm.

Meditation is essentially a vehicle for accessing a higher level of consciousness that is beyond thought, where you are reconnected to your deepest self, your true nature of joy, peace and happiness. When you meditate, you effectively increase your level of self-awareness and you awaken to the things that are beyond thought - love, beauty, peace... This cannot be rationalized intellectually; however it can be experienced when you bring stillness into your mind.

Moreover, meditation does not require effort. As mentioned earlier, it is not about trying to empty your mind. Spiritual leader Deepak Chopra puts it beautifully: "*Meditation is not a way of making your mind quiet. It is a way of entering into the quiet that is already there - buried under the 50 000 thoughts the average person thinks everyday.*"

When you practice meditation, you gain control over your mind, you break the cycle of seeking stimulation from the external world and you learn to draw your state from within. Meditation is truly a transformative experience that can have profound effects not just on your mind, but on virtually every aspect of your life – your body, relationships, health and even your career.

124

Chapter 2 - The Benefits of Meditation

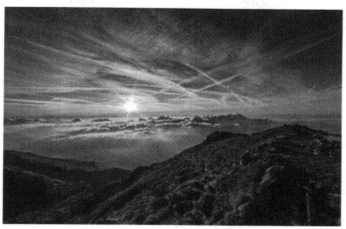

"Meditation more than anything in my life was the biggest ingredient of whatever success I've had."
Ray Dalio

Over the past decade, a vast amount of scientific research has been carried out to investigate the benefits of meditation for the human mind and body. The National Institute of Health has spent over $100 million toward research on meditation, and nowadays it seems like new studies professing the benefits of meditation are emerging everyday.

As a result of the various scientific discoveries on the benefits of meditation, a growing number of hospitals and medical centers are now teaching meditation to patients in order to address various health ailments, relieve pain and fight stress. For example, one famous meditation program called *Mindfulness Based Stress Reduction*, which was created in 1979 by Dr Jon Kabat-Zinn has become so popular that it is now offered in over 200 medical centers around the world.

125

One remarkable example of the effectiveness of meditation for pain relief is shown in a study conducted by Dr Fadel Zeidan at the Wake Forest Medical Center in North Carolina. In the study, 15 people who had never practiced meditation attended four, 20-minute mindfulness meditation classes. The participants' brain activity was examined before and after the training using magnetic resonance imaging. During both scans, they were exposed to a pain-inducing heat device. The results were impressive: After the training, the participant's pain intensity was reduced by about 40% and their pain unpleasantness by around 57%: 80 minutes of meditation was more effective than pain relieving drugs like morphine, which normally reduces pain by about 25%.

Meditation has also become popular in the corporate world, with some leading companies like Google providing meditation classes to their employees to relieve stress, improve focus and boost productivity. The search giant even took it a step further by building a labyrinth to encourage the practice of walking meditation. Moreover, Google is not the only company that is embracing meditation. In fact, other big corporations like Apple, Nike, Yahoo, McKinsey & Co... have all brought meditation to their workplaces in an endeavor to keep employees happy and productive.

Even schools are now adopting meditation to make kids calmer and more focused. Youth meditation program are being installed everywhere in the US, England, Canada and India. In 2014, Educational Psychology Review examined 15 peer-reviewed studies on meditation in schools and concluded that the practice had a myriad of positive effects on students, such as lessened anxiety, increased focus and stronger friendships.

Over 3,000 scientific studies have now been conducted on the benefits of meditation and the truth is practicing meditation has so many benefits that I could not list them all in this book. So here are 53 noteworthy benefits of developing a regular meditation practice:

Health Benefits

- Lowers blood pressure more effectively than medication
- Relieves pain more effectively than morphine
- Slows the progression of HIV
- Helps prevent fibromyalgia and arthritis
- Reduces risk of Alzheimer's
- Reduces risk of heart disease and stroke
- Provides rest deeper than sleep
- Helps recover from addiction
- Improves cardiovascular function
- Relieves irritable bowel syndrome
- Increases energy levels
- Slows down the aging process
- Improves athletic performance
- Improves quality of sleep
- Improves fertility
- Decreases muscle tension
- Improves skin tone
- Increases air flow to the lungs
- Boosts the immune system
- Reduces inflammation

Mental and Emotional Benefits

- Improves attention, focus and ability to work under pressure
- Helps manage ADHD
- Improves intelligence and memory
- Improves critical thinking and decision-making
- Fosters creativity
- Slows down cognitive decline
- Builds composure and calm in all situations
- Increases brain connectivity
- Improves mental strength
- Improves sex life
- Cultivates willpower
- Boosts cognitive function
- Increases grey matter in the hippocampus and frontal areas of the brain
- Helps manage emotional eating
- Promotes good mood
- Improves working memory and executive functioning
- Helps beat depression
- Reduces stress and anxiety
- Improves emotional stability
- Fosters empathy and positive relationships
- Decreases feelings of nervousness
- Reduces social isolation
- Enhances feelings of happiness and vitality
- Improves communication with other people
- Develops a sense of calm and serenity

Spiritual Benefits

- Enhances self-awareness
- Fosters peace of mind, happiness and joy
- Increases self-acceptance
- Boosts self-compassion
- Increases self-esteem
- Develops intuition
- Builds wisdom
- Increases capacity for love

→ Available on Amazon

Preview of
The Mindfulness Beginner's Bible

→ Available on Amazon

Chapter 1 - What is mindfulness?

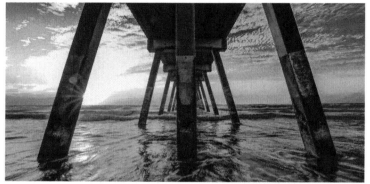

"Life is a dance. Mindfulness is witnessing that dance."

Amit Ray

Have you ever started eating a packet of chips and then suddenly realize that there is nothing left? This is one example of mindlessness that most of us experience on a daily basis. We, as humans often get so absorbed in our thoughts that we fail to experience what is happening right in front of us.

In modern society, most of us suffer from a condition called compulsive thinking. We have this hysterical inner voice that is constantly jumping from one thought to the next, obsessing about every little detail that could go wrong, complaining, comparing and criticizing everything and everyone. Sadly, most of us have become hostages to the whims of our minds, to the point where we even identify with the mind, thinking that we are our thoughts, when in reality we are the awareness behind our thoughts.

The moment you start observing your thoughts without identifying with them, you enter a higher level of consciousness beyond the mind and you reconnect with your true Self – the eternal part of you that is beyond the transient, ever-wavering physical realm.

Take a few seconds right now and become mindful of your hands. Feel the warmth that emanates from them. Rest your attention on every sensation in your hands. Feel your blood pulsing through them. Become one with your hands and notice the subtle tingling sensation as you become aware of them.

If you did this little exercise, I bet you noticed your mind becoming a bit more still. When you rest your attention on your body, you are living actively in the now. Awareness of the body instantly grounds you in the present moment and helps you awaken to a vast realm of consciousness beyond the mind, where all the things that truly matter - love, beauty, peace, creativity and joy - arise from.

Research has shown that we spend up to 50% of the time inside our heads - a state of mindlessness where we are continuously consumed by the chaotic impulses of our minds that are constantly thinking, ruminating the past and worrying about the future. Sadly, most people go through life in a walking haze, never really experiencing the present moment, which is our most precious asset.

Mindfulness is about being fully immersed into your inner and outer experience of the present moment. One of the best definitions of mindfulness is provided by the mindfulness teacher Jon Kabat-Zinn: *"Mindfulness means paying attention in a particular way; On purpose, in the present moment, and non-judgmentally."*

Jon Kabat-Zinn breaks down mindfulness into its fundamental components: In mindfulness, our attention is held...

On purpose

Paying attention on purpose means intentionally directing your awareness. It goes beyond merely being aware of something. It means deliberately focusing your conscious awareness wherever you choose to, instead of being carried away in the perpetual storm of your thoughts.

Secondly, our attention is plunged...

In the Present Moment

The mind's natural tendency is to wander away from the present and get lost in the past or the future. Mindfulness requires being in complete non-resistance to the present moment.

Finally, our attention is held...

Non judgmentally

In mindfulness there is no judgment, there is no labeling, there is no resistance and there is no attachment. You simply observe your thoughts, feelings and sensations as they arise without ever energizing with them. As soon as you realize that you are not your thoughts, but the observer behind your

132

thoughts, they will immediately lose power over your.

Mindfulness goes beyond basic awareness of your present experience. You could be aware that you are drinking tea, for example, however mindfully drinking tea looks very different. When you are mindfully drinking tea, you are purposefully aware of the entire process of drinking tea – you feel the warmth of the cup, the subtleties in smell and taste of the tea, the sensation of heat as you press your lips against the cup... – you intentionally immerse yourself in every single sensory detail that makes up the experience of drinking tea, to the point where you completely dissolve into the activity.

Mindfulness is about maintaining the intention of being completely plunged into your experience, whether it is drinking tea, breathing or doing the dishes. You can bring mindfulness to virtually any activity in your life.

Chapter 2 - The Power of the Present Moment

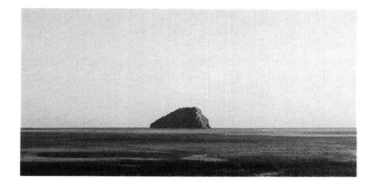

"I have realized that the past and future are real illusions, that they exist in the present, which is what there is and all there is."
Alan Watts

When you think about it, the present moment is the only moment that really exists. The past and the future are merely persistent illusions – the past is obviously over, and the future hasn't happened yet. As the saying goes, *"Tomorrow never comes"*. The future is merely a mental construct that is always around the corner.

Even when you dwell on the past or worry about the future, you're doing so in the present moment. At the end of the day, the present moment is all you and I have, and to spend most of our time outside the present means we are never truly living. Spiritual leader Eckhart Tolle puts it beautifully: *"People don't realize that now is all there ever is; there is no past or future except as memory or anticipation in your mind."*

However, most people spend most of their waking time imprisoned within the walls of their own thoughts, usually in regret of the past or in fear of the future, which are two ways of not living at all.

The present is the only moment in our lives where we have complete control over our destiny. We can decide our course of action only in the now – we can make a new friend, start a new business, get back to the gym, decide to stop smoking... The present is the only moment where your creative power can be exercised; it is the only place where you have full control over your life. Embracing the present moment is the only way to live a happier, healthier and more fulfilling life. As Buddha said, *"The secret of health for both mind and body is not to mourn for the past, worry about the future, or anticipate troubles, but to live in the present moment wisely and earnestly."*

The biggest obstacle that keeps us from living in the present moment is the mind. Embracing mindfulness is a journey that requires practice and dedication, but it is a process that will inevitably lead you to a much happier and more fulfilling life where every moment is lived to the fullest. Here are 8 steps to start living in the present moment:

Practice non-resistance

The first step towards living in the present is learning to live in acceptance. You must learn to accept your life as it is today, rather than wish it was any other way. You must come into complete non-resistance with your current experience of life. By letting go of the hold the past has over you, you free your mind from unproductive thoughts and you reclaim the present moment. As Eckhart Tolle says, *"Accept - then act. Whatever the present moment contains, accept it as if you had chosen it. Always work with it, not against it."*

Focus on the Now

In order to live in the present moment, you must focus on what you are doing in the now, whatever it may be. If you are doing the dishes, then do the dishes. If you're eating dinner, then eat dinner. Don't view the seemingly mundane activities in your life as nuisances that you hurry to get out of the way. These moments are what our lives are made up of, and not being present in them means we are not truly living.

Don't take your thoughts too seriously

Identification with the mind is the root of much unhappiness, disease and misery in the world. Most people have become so identified with their mental chatter that they become slaves to their own compulsive thoughts. Being unable to stop thinking and means we are never living in the present moment. When you learn to observe your thoughts as they come and go without identification, you step away from the chaotic impulses of the mind and you ground yourself in the now.

Meditate

You don't have to meditate to be mindful, but research has shown that engaging in a regular meditation practice has a spillover effect on the rest of your life. When you meditate you essentially carry the state of stillness and awareness that you experience during your meditation session into the rest of your day. Meditation is practice for the rest of your life.

Pay attention to the little things

Notice the seemingly insignificant things around you. Pay attention to nature for example. Notice the greenery around you - be grateful for every tree, every plant, every flower and realize that you could not survive without their presence. Go through your life as if everything is a miracle. From the majestic rising of the sun, to the chirping of birds outside your window, to the fact that your heart is beating every single second – life is truly a miracle to behold when you immerse yourself in the present moment.

Do one thing at a time

Multitasking is the opposite of living in the now. When your attention is divided between several tasks like eating, driving, making a phone call, you cannot fully experience the present moment. Studies have shown that people who multitask take about 50% longer to complete a task with a 50% larger error rate. To be more mindful, you must become a single-tasker. When you're eating, just eat. When you're talking to people, just talk to them. Develop the habit of being completely immersed into whatever you're doing. Not only will you be more efficient, but you'll also be more alive.

Don' try to quiet your mind

Living in the present moment does not require any special effort. The present moment is already at your fingertips. There is no need to expand energy to empty your mind. In mindfulness there is no stress, no struggle and no effort because you are not trying to force anything – you are in complete non-resistance to your current experience of life.

Stop worrying about the future

Worry takes you out of the present moment and in the future into an infinite world of possibilities. You cannot worry about the future and simultaneously live in the present moment. Instead of worrying about things that may or may not happen, spend you time preparing to the best of your ability and let go of the rest. Worrying won't change the future, but it will definitely elevate the cortisol levels in your body and drain you of your vital energy.

→ Available on Amazon

Made in the USA
San Bernardino, CA
09 September 2017